Massachusetts General Hospital

1000 Psychiatry Questions and Annotated Answers

Notice

Medicine is an ever-changing science. As new research and clinical experience broaden our knowledge, changes in treatment and drug therapy are required. The authors and the publisher of this work have checked with sources believed to be reliable in their efforts to provide information that is complete and generally in accord with the standards accepted at the time of publication. However, in view of the possibility of human error or changes in medical sciences, neither the authors nor the publisher nor any other party who has been involved in the preparation or publication of this work warrants that the information contained herein is in every respect accurate or complete, and they disclaim all responsibility for any errors or omissions or for the results obtained from use of the information contained in this work. Readers are encouraged to confirm the information contained herein with other sources. For example and in particular, readers are advised to check the product information sheet included in the package of each drug they plan to administer to be certain that the information contained in this work is accurate and that changes have not been made in the recommended dose or in the contraindications for administration. This recommendation is of particular importance in connection with new or infrequently used drugs.

Massachusetts General Hospital

1000 Psychiatry Questions and Annotated Answers

THEODORE A. STERN, M.D.
Chief, The Avery D. Weisman, M.D., Psychiatry Consultation Service
Massachusetts General Hospital
Professor of Psychiatry, Harvard Medical School
Boston, Massachusetts

JOHN B. HERMAN, M.D.
Director of Clinical Services
Director of Post-Graduate Education, Department of Psychiatry
Massachusetts General Hospital
Medical Director, EAP
Partners HealthCare, Inc.
Assistant Professor of Psychiatry, Harvard Medical School
Boston, Massachusetts

McGraw-Hill
Medical Publishing Division

New York   Chicago   San Francisco   Lisbon
London   Madrid   Mexico City   Milan   New Delhi   San Juan
Seoul   Singapore   Sydney   Toronto

The *McGraw·Hill* Companies

Massachusetts General Hospital 1000 Psychiatry Questions and Annotated Answers

1 2 3 4 5 6 7 8 9 0   DOC/DOC   0 9 8 7 6 5 4

ISBN 0-07-143201-9

This book was set in Berkeley by North Market Street Graphics.
The editors were Marc Strauss and Michelle Watt.
The production supervisor was Catherine Saggese.
Project management was provided by North Market Street Graphics.
The index was prepared by Christine Furry.
RR Donnelley was printer and binder.

This book is printed on acid-free paper.

Cataloging-in-Publication Data for this title is on file at the Library of Congress.

Question and Answer Code Key

The first number inside the parentheses reflects the question number.

The numbers found to the right of the question number indicate which chapter(s) of the *MGH Psychiatry Update and Board Preparation,* 2nd edition will provide supplementary information.

Letters to the right of these references indicate the domain of the question:

c = consultation psychiatry
g = general psychiatry
p = psychopharmacology
d = diagnosis-related
t = treatment-related
f = true-false questions
m = multiple choice question
a = reference: *The MGH Guide to Primary Care Psychiatry,* 2nd edition
d = reference: *Manual of Neurologic Therapeutics,* 5th edition
f = reference: *The MGH Guide to Psychiatry in Primary Care*

The last number inside the parentheses refers to the chapter number in references a, d, or f.

Questions

1. *DSM-IV* criteria for major depressive disorder include each of the following *except*

a. Depressed mood for two or more weeks
b. Disturbance of appetite
c. Panic attacks
d. Psychomotor agitation or retardation
e. Thoughts of death or suicide

2. Each of the following is true about major depressive disorder (MDD) *except*

a. The lifetime risk of MDD in men ranges from 7 to 12%.
b. The lifetime risk of MDD in women ranges from 20 to 25%.
c. More than 50% of patients with MDD receive treatment for their condition.
d. More than 50% of patients treated for MDD are treated by nonpsychiatric physicians.
e. Patients with MDD have generally worse physical and social functioning than those with chronic medical disorders.

3. Each of the following is true about dysthymic disorder *except*

a. The lifetime risk is between 6 and 7% in the general population.
b. The female-to-male ratio is 7:1.
c. Dysthymia is a form of mild, chronic depression.
d. Dysthymia may involve feelings of hopelessness.
e. Recurrent thoughts of death or suicide are present.

4. The side-effect *least* commonly associated with use of selective serotonin reuptake inhibitors (SSRIs) is

a. Dizziness
b. Dry mouth
c. Excessive sweating
d. Nausea
e. Sexual dysfunction

5. Blockade of cholinergic muscarinic receptors by tricyclic antidepressants (TCAs) causes each of the following *except*

a. Blurred vision
b. Constipation
c. Dry mouth
d. Orthostatic hypotension
e. Urinary retention

6. Blockade of which type of receptors is responsible for weight gain, increased appetite, and sedation?

a. Cholinergic muscarinic receptors
b. α_1-adrenergic receptors
c. Histamine H_1 receptors
d. Dopamine receptors
e. None of the above

7. Which of the following is *not* a tricyclic antidepressant?

a. Clomipramine
b. Desipramine
c. Nortriptyline
d. Paroxetine
e. Protriptyline

8. Which of the following is a tetracyclic antidepressant?

a. Amoxapine
b. Doxepin
c. Maprotiline
d. Trimipramine
e. Venlafaxine

9. Which of the following agents is *contraindicated* in the treatment of patients with bulimia?

a. Bupropion
b. Mirtazapine
c. Nefazodone
d. Trazodone
e. Venlafaxine

10. Which statement about bupropion is *false?*

a. Bupropion is contraindicated in patients with seizures.
b. The maximum recommended daily dose is 450 mg/day.
c. The maximum recommended single dose is 150 mg.
d. Blurred vision is a common side effect.
e. Insomnia is a common side effect.

11. Mirtazapine significantly blocks which type of receptors?

a. Cholinergic receptors
b. Histaminic receptors
c. α_1-adrenergic receptors
d. Dopamine receptors
e. None of the above

12. Which of the following statements about phenelzine is *false?*

a. Phenelzine inhibits both monoamine oxidase (MAO) type A and type B.
b. Phenelzine is considered to be a relatively irreversible monoamine oxidase inhibitor (MAOI).
c. Phenelzine, when combined with foods containing tryptophan, can cause a hypertensive crisis.
d. Phenelzine use often causes orthostatic hypotension.
e. Phenelzine use is often associated with weight gain.

13. Which of the following statements about electroconvulsive therapy (ECT) is *false?*

a. ECT involves the application of electrical current to the skull.
b. ECT is relatively contraindicated in the presence of coronary artery disease.
c. Electrical current can be delivered by either sine-wave or brief-pulse current.
d. Side effects of ECT include retrograde and anterograde amnesia.
e. ECT is absolutely contraindicated in the presence of increased intracranial pressure.

14. Which of the following statements about antidepressants is *true?*

a. Most patients show a robust response in the first two months of antidepressant treatment.
b. Two to four weeks of antidepressant treatment is an adequate interval to determine a response.
c. One should only use one antidepressant at a time.
d. Phenelzine should not be started within five weeks after discontinuation of fluoxetine.
e. All antidepressants are equally effective.

15. Which of the following statements about depression is *false?*

a. The risk of relapse after antidepressant withdrawal only abates after at least two months of sustained treatment.
b. Patients who have had at least one episode of major depression are likely to suffer a recurrence.
c. A risk factor for recurrent depression is a long duration (i.e., more than two years) of an index episode.
d. Antidepressants in dosages comparable to those used during the acute phase have been effective in preventing recurrent depressive episodes.
e. SSRIs can be safely combined with tricyclic antidepressants (TCAs) to treat depression.

16. Which of the following statements about suicide is *false?*

a. Suicide is the eighth-leading cause of death in the U.S.
b. Suicide attempts occur 18 to 20 times more often than completed suicides.
c. Survival of a premeditated attempt reduces one's risk for a repeat attempt.
d. The patient who has no hopes for the future is at risk for suicide.
e. Lack of outpatient providers, family, or friends may elevate the potential risk for suicide.

17. Which of the following statements about suicide is *false?*

a. Individuals over 65 years old are more likely to commit suicide than are younger individuals.
b. The elderly account for 20% of all completed suicides.
c. Among individuals between the ages of 15 and 24, suicide has become the leading cause of death.
d. Four times more men than women complete suicide.
e. Major depressive disorder accounts for roughly 50% of suicides.

18. Which of the following statements about suicide is *false?*

a. Major depressive disorder accounts for more suicides than do psychotic disorders.

b. Alcohol and drug dependence are responsible for more suicides than psychotic disorders.

c. Anxiety disorders, especially panic disorder, are increasingly reported among suicide victims.

d. Divorced adults are at greater risk for suicide than are those who are widowed.

e. Unemployment is associated with as many as one-third to one-half of completed suicides.

19. Which of the following statements about the evaluation of a potentially suicidal patient is *false?*

a. Medication is indicated for the uncooperative and potentially suicidal patient.

b. Physical restraints may be needed for patients who cannot reliably contract for safety.

c. The potential means for self-harm must be removed from the reach of patients at risk.

d. Patients being evaluated for suicide must be detained until their risk for suicide has been assessed.

e. The evaluation of suicidal risk in the potentially suicidal patient takes precedence over the desire of the patient for privacy and confidentiality.

20. Which of the following is *not* a feature that distinguishes pathological anxiety from "normal" anxiety?

a. Distress with a minimal relation to an external cause

b. A high level of discomfort and severity of symptoms

c. Persistence of symptoms over time

d. Development of disabling behavioral strategies

e. Disorientation

21. Stimulation of which of the following structures can generate panic attacks?

a. The amygdala

b. The locus coeruleus

c. The anterior cingulate gyrus

d. The median raphe

e. The left caudate nucleus

22. The locus coeruleus is the major source of innervation of which of the brain's neurotransmitters?

a. Serotonin
b. Dopamine
c. Norepinephrine
d. Gamma-aminobutyric acid
e. Glutamate

23. Approximately what percentage of individuals in the U.S. experience pathologic anxiety over the course of their lifetime?

a. Less than 5
b. 5
c. 10
d. 25
e. 50

24. Which of the following statements about panic disorder (PD) is *false?*

a. PD leads to a perceived deterioration in physical and mental health.
b. PD leads to an increase in alcohol abuse.
c. PD leads to an increase in marital problems.
d. PD leads to an increase in suicide attempts.
e. PD leads to an increase in ulcerative colitis.

25. Roughly what percentage of patients with atypical chest pain and normal findings on cardiac catheterization have panic disorder (PD)?

a. Less than 5
b. 5
c. 10
d. 25
e. 50

26. Which of the following is *not* associated with an organic anxiety syndrome, as opposed to a primary anxiety disorder?

a. Onset of symptoms after the age of 35
b. Lack of a personal or family history of an anxiety disorder
c. A childhood history of separation anxiety
d. Lack of avoidance behavior
e. Poor response to anti-panic agents

27. Medications associated with anxiety-like symptoms include each of the following *except*

a. Corticosteroids
b. Thyroid hormone
c. Theophylline
d. Sympathomimetics
e. Beta-blockers

28. Medical conditions that may precipitate anxiety symptoms include each of the following *except*

a. Diabetes
b. Thyroid dysfunction
c. Osteoporosis
d. Seizure disorder
e. Chronic obstructive pulmonary disease (COPD)

29. Which of the following is *not* typical of panic disorder?

a. Onset in the third or fourth decade of life
b. A chronic or recurrent course
c. Occurrence in women more than men
d. The presence of four or more symptoms
e. Successful treatment with high-potency benzodiazepines and cognitive-behavioral therapy

30. Which of the following is a syndrome characterized by discrete episodes of intense anxiety that is associated with at least four symptoms of autonomic arousal and that develops rapidly and peaks within 10 minutes?

a. Generalized anxiety disorder
b. Panic disorder
c. Obsessive-compulsive disorder
d. Post-traumatic stress disorder
e. Social phobia

31. A syndrome with excessive worry or anxiety in the absence of or out of proportion to situational factors or discrete episodes of anxiety that typically lasts over six months is most likely to be diagnosed as

a. Generalized anxiety disorder
b. Panic disorder
c. Obsessive-compulsive disorder
d. Post-traumatic stress disorder
e. Social phobia

32. A syndrome involving prior exposure to an event involving the threat of death, injury, or harm to oneself or others is

a. Generalized anxiety disorder
b. Panic disorder
c. Obsessive-compulsive disorder
d. Post-traumatic stress disorder
e. Social phobia

33. The only tricyclic antidepressant (TCA) thought to be effective in the treatment of obsessive-compulsive disorder (OCD) is

a. Nortriptyline
b. Amitriptyline
c. Desipramine
d. Clomipramine
e. Protriptyline

34. Which statement about benzodiazepines is *true?*

a. Oxazepam is faster-acting than clonazepam.
b. Oxazepam is longer-lasting than clonazepam.
c. Clorazepate is faster-acting than oxazepam.
d. Alprazolam is more potent than clonazepam.
e. Lorazepam is less potent than clorazepate.

35. Which of the following benzodiazepines *lacks* significant metabolites?

a. Oxazepam
b. Chlordiazepoxide
c. Clorazepate
d. Flurazepam
e. Diazepam

36. Which of the following is the longest-acting benzodiazepine?

a. Alprazolam
b. Clorazepate
c. Chlordiazepoxide
d. Lorazepam
e. Oxazepam

37. Side effects of benzodiazepines include each of the following *except*

a. Sedation
b. Behavioral disinhibition
c. Ataxia
d. Reduction in the seizure threshold
e. Respiratory depression

38. Discontinuation of benzodiazepines is often associated with each of the following *except*

a. Nervousness
b. Seizures
c. Insomnia
d. Constipation
e. Irritability

39. Which of the following mental and emotional signs is *not* typical of a response to stress?

a. Lack of concentration
b. Memory lapses
c. Dissociation
d. Anxiety
e. Hostility

40. Physiological signs of acute stress include each of the following *except*

a. Tense muscles
b. Fatigue
c. Palpitations
d. Miosis
e. Dry mouth

41. Techniques often employed to deal with acute stress responses include each of the following *except*

a. Breathing exercises
b. Projection
c. Visualization
d. Meditation
e. Biofeedback

42. Stress responses may result from each of the following *except*

a. Benzodiazepine withdrawal
b. Physical ailments
c. Job insecurity
d. Marital discord
e. Dissatisfaction in the workplace

43. Evaluation of chronic stress includes each of the following *except*

a. A determination as to whether bodily complaints follow an anatomic distribution
b. Search for personal social and work-related tasks as sources of stress
c. An assessment of the individual's coping skills
d. Review of the patient's insurance benefits
e. Assessment of whether the patient's current stresses exceed his or her coping resources

44. Which of the following is *not* consistent with a stress response?

a. Elevated digital skin temperature
b. High electromyogram (EMG) activity of the frontalis muscle
c. Current medical symptoms in the absence of a clear medical explanation
d. New onset of symptoms temporally related to current life stressors
e. Tense muscles, palpitations, and diaphoresis

45. Relaxation training may include each of the following *except*

a. Progressively tensing and relaxing large muscle groups
b. Diaphragmatic breathing
c. Hypnotic inductions or mindfulness meditation
d. Inspiratory-expiratory breathing cycles of five to seven seconds in duration
e. Cognitive restructuring

46. Which of the following statements about alcohol use and abuse is *false?*

a. Alcoholism causes 80% of hepatic cirrhosis.
b. Patients injured while under the influence of alcohol fill 33% of American trauma beds.
c. Alcohol-related problems are the third-leading cause of death in the U.S.
d. Alcohol dependence is defined as the excessive and recurrent use of alcohol despite medical, psychological, social, and/or economic problems.
e. Alcohol abuse spans the continuum from brief episodes of excessive drinking to chronic patterns that produce significant problems but never progress to psychological or physical dependence.

47. Which of the following statements about alcohol abuse is *false?*

a. Alcohol abuse cannot be diagnosed in the presence of major depression.
b. With alcohol abuse, recurrent use of alcohol in physically dangerous situations can occur.
c. With alcohol abuse, continued use of alcohol despite recurrent social or interpersonal problems may occur.
d. Alcohol abuse is frequently associated with motor vehicle accidents.
e. Alcohol abuse occurs along a continuum from brief episodes of excessive drinking to chronic patterns of use.

48. What percentage of alcohol abusers also have at least one other psychiatric diagnosis?

a. 10 to 15%
b. 25 to 30%
c. 35 to 40%
d. 45 to 50%
e. Over 50%

49. What percentage of mentally ill individuals abuse alcohol or other drugs?

a. 10 to 15%
b. 25 to 30%
c. 35 to 40%
d. 45 to 50%
e. Over 50%

50. Which of the following is *not* part of the CAGE criteria to screen for alcohol abuse?

a. Have you ever had a drink first thing in the morning?
b. Have you ever felt bad about your drinking?
c. Have you ever felt you should cut down on your drinking?
d. Have people annoyed you by criticizing your drinking?
e. Have you felt it would be easy to stop drinking?

51. The presence of certain medical disorders heightens the probability of an alcohol-use disorder. Which of the following does *not* suggest an alcohol-use disorder?

a. Peripheral neuropathy
b. Gastrointestinal bleeding
c. Hypothyroidism
d. Cardiomyopathy
e. Pancreatitis

52. Which of the following statements about screening tests for alcohol abuse is *false?*

a. The Alcohol Use Disorders Identification Test (AUDIT) is a 10-item questionnaire developed by the World Health Organization (WHO) for early detection of patients with alcohol problems in the primary care setting.
b. The CAGE questionnaire is a four-item screen for alcoholism.
c. One or more positive responses on the CAGE test correlates with significant alcohol-related problems.
d. The Michigan Alcoholism Screening Test (MAST) is a 25-item questionnaire.
e. The MAST is more accurate than the CAGE for detection of alcoholism.

53. What percentage of alcoholics are depressed when admitted for detoxification?

a. 10 to 15%
b. 25 to 30%
c. 35 to 40%
d. 45 to 50%
e. Over 50%

54. Which of the following benzodiazepines is *most* commonly used for detoxification of the alcoholic patient with normal liver function?

a. Oxazepam
b. Chlordiazepoxide
c. Alprazolam
d. Temazepam
e. Midazolam

55. Which of the following is *usually* recommended for an alcohol-abusing individual (with significant liver disease) undergoing detoxification?

a. Chlordiazepoxide
b. Diazepam
c. Lorazepam
d. Flurazepam
e. Clorazepate

56. Which of the following statements about naltrexone is *false?*

a. It is often given in doses of 50 mg/day.
b. It is an opiate agonist.
c. It seems to work best in a patient who describes intense craving.
d. It is contraindicated in a patient with acute hepatitis.
e. It is contraindicated in a patient with liver failure.

57. Which of the following statements about disulfiram is *false?*

a. Doses of 250 mg/day can produce tachycardia and dyspnea if the alcohol-abusing patient drinks alcohol.
b. It is no better than placebo in producing continuous abstinence from alcohol.
c. It inhibits alcohol metabolism and leads to elevated levels of acetaldehyde.
d. It inhibits dopamine beta hydroxylase.
e. Its use does not require monitoring of liver function.

58. Which of the following statements about migraine headaches is *false?*

a. Ninety percent of afflicted individuals have their first attack by age 40.
b. A family history is present in up to 90% of migraine sufferers.
c. After puberty, migraines are more common in women than in men.
d. The prevalence of migraines in females is approximately five percent.
e. The prevalence of migraine headaches is greater in boys than in girls.

59. Which of the following statements about patients with cluster headaches is *false?*

a. A family history of cluster headaches is usually present.
b. The ratio of men to women is 5:1.
c. The estimated percent of patients with cluster headaches is between 0.08 and 0.4 percent.
d. A higher incidence of duodenal ulceration is present.
e. A higher incidence of elevated gastric acid levels is present.

60. Which of the following statements about migraine headaches is *false?*

a. A migraine headache is usually bilateral.
b. Migraine headaches are usually severe and throbbing.
c. Migraines are often experienced behind the eyes.
d. Photophobia and sonophobia are common with migraines.
e. Nausea and vomiting are common features of migraines.

61. Which of the following statements about cluster headaches is *false?*

a. Cluster headaches are the most painful type of recurrent headache.
b. Stereotyped attacks are usually present.
c. Cluster headaches come on slowly and peak in 45 to 60 minutes.
d. Injected conjunctiva, nasal blockage, and facial flushing on the side of the headache are common.
e. Ptosis and miosis on the side of the pain are common.

Questions 62 to 73 are *true-false* questions.

62. Tension headaches may be concentrated in the frontal, nuchal, or occipital area.

63. Intracranial aneurysms are rarely responsible for headache unless they rupture.

64. Arteriovenous malformations (AVMs) commonly cause pain before they rupture.

65. Headaches in response to subarachnoid hemorrhage are typically explosive in nature.

66. Vomiting is uncommon with rupture of intracranial arteriovenous malformations (AVMs).

67. Migraine headaches usually start during the teenage years.

68. Tension headaches usually begin before age 10.

69. Migraine headaches may be precipitated by eating chocolate and by drinking alcoholic beverages.

70. Bright lights may induce a migraine headache.

71. Cluster headaches often occur during the night or one to two hours after going to sleep.

72. Patients with cluster headaches, unlike those with migraine headaches, prefer to pace during an attack.

73. Papilledema is a feature of pseudotumor cerebri.

74. Which is *not* an acute treatment for migraines?
a. Sumatriptan
b. Aspirin
c. Ibuprofen
d. Fiorinal
e. Propranolol

75. Which is *not* a prophylactic treatment for migraine?
a. Verapamil
b. Propranolol
c. Sodium valproate
d. Sumatriptan
e. Phenytoin

76. Which is *not* a treatment for cluster headache?

a. 100% nasal oxygen
b. Sublingual or parenteral ergots
c. Steroids
d. Indomethacin
e. Propranolol

77. Parasomnias include each of the following *except*

a. Sleepwalking
b. Enuresis
c. Bruxism
d. Restless legs
e. Night terrors

78. Which of the following statements about prolonged sleep latency is *false?*

a. It is defined by an inability to fall asleep in less than 30 minutes.
b. It can be diagnosed by use of polysomnography.
c. It is commonly seen in insomnia.
d. It is associated with the immediate onset of rapid eye movement (REM) sleep.
e. It is often treated with hypnotic agents.

79. Parameters typically monitored during polysomnography include each of the following *except*

a. Muscle activity
b. Respiratory rate
c. Electroencephalogram
d. Skin temperature
e. Activity of eye muscles

80. Which of the following antidepressants is thought to be the *least* sedating?

a. Trazodone
b. Nortriptyline
c. Paroxetine
d. Doxepin
e. Bupropion

81. Which of the following statements about hypersomnia is *false?*

a. It is characterized by prolonged episodes of sleep.
b. It can be documented by testing in a sleep laboratory.
c. It may result from sleep apnea.
d. It rarely occurs during conversation or while carrying out potentially hazardous activities.
e. It is often marked by excessive daytime sleepiness.

82. Current treatments for sleep apnea include each of the following *except*

a. Weight loss
b. Avoidance of alcohol
c. Continuous positive airway pressure
d. Tonsillectomy
e. Uvulopalatopharyngoplasty

83. Loud snoring is commonly *present* in patients with which of the following?

a. Parasomnias
b. Narcolepsy
c. Sleep apnea
d. Congestive heart failure
e. Chronic obstructive pulmonary disease

84. Common associated features of sleep apnea include each of the following *except*

a. Irritability
b. Impotence
c. Headache
d. Pulmonary hypertension
e. Two to four episodes of apnea or hypopnea per hour of sleep

85. Which of the following is *not* part of the tetrad of symptoms in narcolepsy?

a. Sleepwalking
b. Sleep attacks
c. Cataplexy
d. Sleep paralysis
e. Hypnagogic hallucinations

For the following questions (86 to 90), match up the correct choices in each column.

86. Sleepwalking
87. Sleep paralysis
88. Cataplexy
89. Sleep attacks
90. Hypnagogic hallucinations

a. Irresistible, usually brief episodes of sleep, that may occur several times each day
b. A condition involving the sudden loss of muscle tone without impaired consciousness usually triggered by emotion
c. A complete loss of muscle tone in the absence of sleep
d. A non-REM sleep state involving ambulation
e. Visual hallucinations that occur while falling asleep

For the following questions (91 to 95), match up the correct choices in each column.

91. Bruxism
92. Central sleep apnea
93. Night terrors
94. Restless legs syndrome
95. Nocturnal myoclonus

a. A condition in which no respiratory effort is made until arousal supervenes
b. A condition in which achy feelings or paresthesias in the legs appear at night
c. Brief involuntary leg movements that occur every 20 to 40 seconds during sleep
d. A dramatic state of autonomic arousal during non-REM sleep
e. A parasomnia usually involving grinding of the teeth

96. Causes of dizziness include each of the following *except*

a. Vertebro-basilar episodes
b. Cuprolithiasis
c. Perilymph fistula
d. Labyrinthitis
e. Craniopharyngioma

97. Central causes of dizziness include each of the following *except*

a. Multiple sclerosis
b. Cerebello-pontine angle tumors
c. Brainstem transient ischemic attacks
d. Dysfunction of the eighth cranial nerve
e. Labyrinthitis

Questions 98 to 100 are *true-false* questions.

98. Peripheral causes of vertigo result from the stimulation of the semicircular canals, the utricle, and the saccule.

99. Central causes of vertigo include dysfunction of the eighth cranial nerve, the vestibular nuclei, the brainstem, and their central connections.

100. Ménière's syndrome can be associated with loss of consciousness that is preceded by severe vertigo and vomiting.

101. Systemic causes of vertigo include each of the following *except*

a. Postural hypotension
b. Use of antihypertensives
c. Use of analgesics
d. Multiple sclerosis
e. Multiple sensory deficits

102. Which of the following statements about fatigue is *false?*

a. It is a symptom with different meanings, causes, and physical manifestations.
b. It may become chronic and disabling.
c. It is associated with higher rates of anxiety and depression.
d. It may be a normal response to exercise.
e. It is an uncommon complaint in ambulatory medical settings.

103. Medical causes of fatigue include each of the following *except*

a. Hypothyroidism
b. Parkinson's disease
c. Chemotherapy
d. Thrombocytopenia
e. Hepatitis

104. Which of the following statements is *false?*

a. Patients with multiple unexplained physical complaints make up a significant proportion of primary care populations.
b. Patients with hypochondriasis lie about their symptoms or feign physical symptoms to simulate disease.
c. Somatoform disorders include hypochondriasis and somatization disorder.
d. Somatoform pain disorder is more common than somatization disorder.
e. Somatization is the tendency to experience or report bodily symptoms that have no physiologic explanation and to misattribute symptoms to disease.

105. *La belle indifférence,* or emotional indifference, may be a feature of

a. Right parietal lesions
b. Hypochondriasis
c. Somatoform pain disorder
d. Body dysmorphic disorder
e. Somatization disorder

106. Which of the following statements about hypochondriacal patients is *false?*

a. They tend to describe symptoms in an obsessive and all-inclusive way.
b. They tend to focus on gastrointestinal and cardiovascular symptoms.
c. They often make friends based on common medical problems.
d. They fear occult disease.
e. Their symptoms are often alleviated by use of pimozide.

107. Systemic medical disorders to be considered when a patient presents with medically unexplained complaints include each of the following *except*

a. Brucellosis
b. Hyperparathyroidism
c. Acute intermittent porphyria
d. Systemic lupus erythematosus
e. Temporal lobe epilepsy

Questions 108 to 112 are *true-false* questions.

108. Anxiety disorders occur in a majority of patients with hypochondriasis.

109. Conversion disorder involves a change in voluntary motor or sensory function that suggests a neurologic condition but defies explanation.

110. The incidence of personality disorders among patients with somatoform disorders is low.

111. The triad of bodily preoccupation, disease fear, and disease conviction is crucial to the diagnosis of somatization disorder.

112. Hypochondriacal patients typically have two gastrointestinal symptoms, one pseudoneurological symptom, four pain symptoms, and one sexual symptom.

113. Which of the following is *not* a criterion for conversion disorder?
a. The patient's symptoms are not intentionally produced.
b. The patient's symptoms are presumed to be associated with psychological feelings.
c. The patient's symptoms are a culturally-sanctioned response to stress.
d. The patient may experience a change in voluntary motor function.
e. The symptoms may present as a single episode or as recurrent episodes.

114. Which of the following is *not* a criterion for somatization disorder?
a. The patient's symptoms are intentionally feigned.
b. The patient's symptoms begin by age 30.
c. The symptoms cannot be caused by drugs.
d. The symptoms are not fully explained by a known physical disorder.
e. The symptoms experienced include gastrointestinal pain, sexual disorders, and pseudoneurological symptoms.

115. Treatment of hypochondriasis may include each of the following *except*
a. Scheduling of regular brief appointments
b. Performance of a physical exam
c. Provision of accurate information about objective signs
d. Recommendations of benign interventions; for example, exercise
e. Diligent investigation of subjective complaints

116. Symptoms commonly experienced by those with chronic fatigue syndrome include each of the following *except*

a. Tender cervical or axillary lymph nodes
b. Sore throat
c. Muscle pain
d. Unrefreshing sleep
e. Abdominal discomfort

117. Symptoms commonly experienced by those with chronic fatigue syndrome include each of the following *except*

a. Self-reported impairment in short-term memory or concentration significant enough to cause substantial reduction in activity
b. Multi-joint pain without swelling or redness
c. Post-exertional malaise of more than 24 hours
d. Dizziness
e. Muscle pain

118. Which of the following statements about chronic fatigue syndrome is *false?*

a. Chronic fatigue syndrome is a homogeneous disorder.
b. Chronic fatigue syndrome is a syndrome defined by consensus.
c. Chronic fatigue syndrome has a social meaning with support from lobbies and support groups.
d. No specific virus has been established as the cause of chronic fatigue syndrome.
e. Chronic fatigue syndrome has symptoms similar to those of fibromyalgia.

119. Principles of medical evaluation in the treatment of chronic fatigue syndrome include each of the following *except*

a. Educate the patient about the role of inactivity in promoting fatigue.
b. Set improved function as the goal.
c. Defer requests for permanent disability.
d. Consider serious and treatable diagnoses during the evaluation.
e. Delay prescriptions for antidepressants until at least two months of symptoms have been present.

120. General approaches to the patient with multiple environmental allergies include each of the following *except*

a. Building an alliance with the patient
b. Avoiding debates about the validity of clinical ecology
c. Setting achievable goals that are specific and measurable
d. Considering referral to an occupational and environmental medicine specialist
e. Administering conventional medicines while monitoring for pupillary diameter after exposure

121. Which of the following statements about multiple environmental allergies is *false?*

a. No specific symptom pattern defines the disorder.
b. No diagnostic laboratory tests exist for this syndrome.
c. Treatment is directed at improving function.
d. Physical examination of the patient is not generally required.
e. Strategies to reduce stress should be encouraged.

122. Which of the following statements about irritable bowel syndrome (IBS) is *false?*

a. It is characterized by abdominal pain.
b. It is characterized by altered stool form.
c. It is characterized by abdominal bloating.
d. It is characterized by the perception of incomplete evacuation.
e. It is characterized by rectal bleeding.

123. Which of the following statements about irritable bowel syndrome (IBS) is *false?*

a. A majority of patients with IBS will have an Axis I psychiatric disorder during their lifetime.
b. IBS patients who seek care tend to be heavy users of health care services.
c. IBS patients who seek care tend to have elevated levels of anxiety, depression, and somatization.
d. IBS is a diagnosis of exclusion.
e. IBS is not associated with a history of physical or sexual abuse.

124. Which of the following psychiatric diagnoses is *least* likely to be found in patients with IBS?

a. Panic disorder
b. Major depressive disorder
c. Somatization disorder
d. Post-traumatic stress disorder
e. Conversion disorder

125. Which of the following statements about independent disability evaluations is *false?*

a. The purpose of the evaluation is to assess the patient's claim.
b. Corroboration of information from other sources is sought.
c. Information obtained in the course of the evaluation is not confidential.
d. Payment for the evaluation comes from the patient, usually through a health insurer.
e. Transference and counter-transference issues are active during the evaluation.

126. Which of the following statements about clinical evaluations related to disability is *false?*

a. Certification of disability may remove a patient from the workplace permanently.
b. The physician may ultimately be called on to justify his or her assessment in court.
c. Inaccurate certification that a patient is no longer disabled can create a risk of harm to the patient and to the patient's co-workers.
d. Generally, a monetary issue is involved when a statement of disability is requested.
e. Typically, the physician neither relies on the patient's report nor acts as the patient's advocate.

Questions 127 to 133 are *true-false* questions.

127. The presence of a psychiatric diagnosis does not automatically confirm disability.

128. An assessment of disability is an assessment of functional capacity.

129. Details of childhood abuse and intimate sexual details are often necessary to provide a clear picture in a report of disability status.

130. Assessment of work-related activities includes determination of the ability to make decisions without immediate supervision.

131. Psychological and neuropsychological testing is rarely helpful or necessary in determining the level of function, the nature of an illness, or the presence of malingering.

132. Your obligation to the patient is to certify disability only when it is appropriate and to return the patient to work only when it is safe to do so.

133. Provision of a job description and the nature of the job's essential function is not a key element of the psychiatric disability evaluation report.

134. Which of the following statements about denial is *false?*
a. Denial often stems from fear of illness and its consequences.
b. Even highly functional adults use denial to cope with anxiety or fear.
c. Denial may be either adaptive or maladaptive.
d. Denial represents an abnormal response to an acute stress such as life-threatening illness.
e. Patients may deny to protect their physicians from feelings of impotence or grief.

Questions 135 to 137 are *true-false* questions.

135. A patient may be noncompliant with a physician's recommendations without being in denial.

136. Anosognosia, or unawareness of a neurologic deficit, stems from left-sided parietal lesions.

137. Bilateral occipital lesions can produce denial of blindness.

138. Strategies for managing denial include each of the following *except*

a. Avoid power struggles and threats.
b. Support the patient's wish to get a second opinion.
c. Listen to the patient's point of view and present your own viewpoint.
d. Encourage the patient to engage in activities of coping with illness that are not harmful.
e. Avoid use of psychotropics; instead allow the patient to resolve his or her dilemma at his or her own pace.

Questions 139 to 144 are *true-false* questions.

139. Elderly persons and their families tend to over-report their symptoms and blame them on advancing age.

140. Obstacles to interviewing the geriatric patient include cognitive decline, vague complaints, and sensory impairments.

141. Acute medical or psychiatric illness often presents differently in older patients compared with younger patients.

142. Depression, dementia, and psychosis can be overlooked when they are erroneously attributed to a medical condition.

143. Geriatric syndromes are problem complexes that combine or cross over multiple organ systems.

144. Measures of activities of daily living (ADLs) are useful in the assessment of functional independence of patients.

145. Which of the following is *not* generally considered to be a basic activity of daily living?

a. Dressing
b. Feeding
c. Toileting
d. Bathing
e. Shopping

Questions 146 to 148 are *true-false* questions.

146. The Geriatric Depression Scale (GDS) has been used widely in primary care settings, but it is invalid if cognitive impairment is present.

147. The Mini Mental State Examination (MMSE) accurately assesses and screens for dysfunction of the parietal, temporal, and frontal lobes.

148. Testing for serial sevens on the MMSE assesses cognitive function and recall.

149. The prevalence of major depressive disorder in the oncologic population is approximately

a. Two percent
b. Five to eight percent
c. 12 to 15%
d. 20 to 23%
e. Greater than 30%

150. Which of the following statements about psychological responses to cancer is *false?*

a. Worrying enough to seek medical advice about a physical symptom and the possibility of having cancer is adaptive.
b. Hypervigilance and an all-consuming preoccupation with the resulting diagnosis constitutes an abnormal response.
c. Patients may initially deny or not believe the diagnosis of cancer.
d. A variably depressed mood in the first month after the diagnosis is abnormal.
e. Complete denial of the diagnosis prevents the patient from considering responsible or reasonable choices.

151. Lethargy is a well-known side-effect of each of the following drugs used to treat cancer *except*

a. Aminoglutethimide
b. L-asparaginase
c. Vincristine
d. Interkeukin-2 (IL-2)
e. Ifosfamide

152. Which of the following drugs used to treat cancer is a hormonal therapy?

a. Procarbazine
b. 5-fluouricil
c. Paclitaxel
d. Tamoxifen
e. Interferon

153. Common neuropsychiatric side-effects of corticosteroids include each of the following *except*

a. Insomnia
b. Depression
c. Mania
d. Emotional lability
e. Complex partial seizures

154. Akathisia may result from each of the following agents *except*

a. Perphenazine
b. Prochlorperazine
c. Aminoglutethimide
d. Metoclopramide
e. Droperidol

155. Which of the following statements about hypercalcemia is *false?*

a. Hypercalcemia causes lethargy.
b. Hypercalcemia causes anorexia.
c. Hypercalcemia causes tetany.
d. Hypercalcemia causes impaired concentration.
e. Hypercalcemia is associated with metastatic disease.

156. Common causes of delirium in patients with cancer include each of the following *except*

a. Use of opiates and anticholinergic medications
b. Electrolyte imbalance
c. Hypoxia
d. Psychological reactions to the diagnosis of cancer
e. Metastatic lesions in the brain

157. Which of the following statements about paraneoplastic syndromes is *false?*

a. Paraneoplastic syndromes are associated with increased ADH secretion and hyponatremia.
b. Paraneoplastic syndromes are associated with increased parathyroid hormone.
c. Paraneoplastic syndromes are associated with increased ACTH and Cushing's syndrome.
d. Paraneoplastic syndromes are associated with lesions in the cerebral cortex.
e. Paraneoplastic syndromes are associated with delirious states.

158. Treatments for post-chemotherapy nausea and vomiting include each of the following *except*

a. Sumatriptan
b. Ondansetron
c. Dexamethasone
d. Droperidol
e. Prochlorperazine

159. Ondansetron's mechanism of action is thought to include which of the following?

a. Dopaminergic agonism
b. Dopaminergic antagonism
c. Serotonergic agonism
d. Serotonergic antagonism
e. Cholinergic agonism

160. Metaclopramide's mechanism of action is thought to include

a. Dopaminergic agonism
b. Dopaminergic antagonism
c. Serotonergic agonism
d. Serotonergic antagonism
e. Cholinergic agonism

161. Palliative care involves each of the following *except*

a. Provision of symptom control
b. Maintenance or repair of family and other interpersonal relationships
c. Maintenance of day-to-day activities necessary for sustaining a comforting home environment
d. Attendance to spiritual concerns
e. Facilitating the end of life with the use of narcotics

Questions 162 to 175 are *true-false* questions.

162. When receiving palliative care, continued aggressive treatment is not clinically or ethically appropriate for the terminally ill.

163. Palliation is treatment aimed primarily at reducing suffering and maximizing quality of life.

164. Hospice care is usually delivered by a multidisciplinary team at the patient's home.

165. Hospice care is generally indicated for the patient who is expected to survive more than six months.

166. The amount of information provided to an adult patient with terminal illness is determined by the patient's spouse.

167. Referral to a hospice means that the physician is giving up on the patient.

168. Patients who are dying secondary to a terminal illness should be forced to eat and drink.

169. While receiving palliative care, persistent physical symptoms may contribute greatly to the emergence and persistence of psychological symptoms.

170. The experience of dying stirs strong feelings in most terminally ill patients and their families.

171. Symptoms in terminally ill patients that are subthreshold for a formal diagnosis of a mental disorder but that cause substantial suffering—for example, depression—should be treated aggressively.

172. The neuropsychiatric complications of terminal illness are commonly recognized and treated.

173. Depression and anxiety are universal among terminally ill patients and are an appropriate part of the experience of dying.

174. Depression has been estimated to occur in up to 15% of patients with a terminal illness.

175. Nearly 30% of patients develop delirium near the end of life.

176. Which of the following statements about psychostimulants is *false?*
a. Psychostimulants have a rapid onset of action.
b. Tolerance may develop requiring a dose increase.
c. Psychostimulants may precipitate agitation or delirium in susceptible patients.
d. Dextroamphetamine should be avoided because of its potential for abuse.
e. Methylphenidate is often prescribed in doses of 2.5 to 20 mg b.i.d. to treat depressive symptoms.

177. Which of the following statements related to the breaking of bad news is *false?*
a. Compassionate communication can make an enormous difference for patients and their families.
b. The physician must bear the consequences of being a messenger of ill tidings.
c. It is best for the physician to sit down with the patient or family member when about to deliver bad news.
d. It is best to give detailed descriptions of the situation when delivering bad news.
e. It is important to concentrate on listening as much as speaking.

Questions 178 to 184 are *true-false* questions.

178. Sometimes the preeminent concern when a patient learns he or she has a serious or life-threatening illness is fear of pain.

179. The physician need not be honest with the patient regarding the severity of the illness.

180. Grief can profoundly affect personal relationships.

181. Although the death of a deeply loved person can cause prolonged grief, this loss is easier to recover from than the loss of someone for whom feelings are complicated or conflicted.

182. Mourning for our offspring is generally more difficult than mourning for our elders or our parents.

183. Physicians should urge parents to get over the loss of a perinatal death as quickly as possible and to get on with attempts to conceive again.

184. Group support after human-made or natural disasters may be as important for the physician as it is for survivors and their relatives.

185. When learning about bad news or of serious or life-threatening illness, which of the following is *not* a common concern of the patient?
a. The physician's belief that the illness was the result of an unhealthy lifestyle
b. The loss of earning capacity and anticipated medical expenses
c. An impending loss of dignity associated with terminal illness
d. Survival until the patient can witness an important milestone
e. Concern about how to tell others about their illness

186. Physicians who deliver bad news about life-threatening illness to a patient often experience each of the following *except*
a. A sense of helplessness
b. A sense of guilt and excessive responsibility
c. Feelings of grief
d. A feeling of catastrophic loss
e. A sense of failure

Questions 187 to 199 are *true-false* questions.

187. Withholding and withdrawing life-sustaining treatment can be both morally and legally permissible.

188. In physician-assisted suicide, the physician administers a medication to a patient to end his or her suffering.

189. Withdrawal of care is psychologically more difficult than is withholding care for a patient.

190. Giving large doses of narcotics to decrease pain or to ease dyspnea, even if it shortens life, is not considered euthanasia.

191. Only a judge can declare a patient to be incompetent.

192. Physicians in general are poor at predicting preference regarding resuscitation.

193. An advance directive documents what should be done when a person becomes incompetent or appoints a surrogate or health care proxy who will judge what the patient would have wanted if he or she were competent.

194. Health care proxies can overrule the decisions of a competent patient.

195. When a patient is alert but incompetent, formal guardianship proceedings must be initiated.

196. A competent adult patient has the legal right to refuse treatment even if that decision will lead to harm.

197. A physician is under no obligation to provide useless or harmful treatment to a patient.

198. A good time to discuss end-of-life treatment decisions with a patient is before a health care crisis occurs.

199. Documentation of discussions about end-of-life decisions should be included in the medical record, because the patient may change his or her mind at some later point in time.

200. Which of the following is *not* a part of the assessment of a patient's preference for treatment at the end of life?

a. An assessment as to whether all symptoms are being aggressively treated.
b. An assessment of the patient's perception of his or her social supports.
c. An assessment of the health care proxy's view on terminal illness.
d. An assessment of the patient's reasons for wanting to be dead.
e. An assessment of the dynamics of the doctor-patient relationship.

201. Which of the following statements about grief is *false?*

a. Grief is usually proportionate to the disruption caused by loss.
b. Seldom does acute grief pose a medical or psychiatric emergency.
c. Grief is an abnormal response to feeling lost and bereaved.
d. Acute grief is the first phase of the bereavement process.
e. Grief is not limited to loss by a death, though it may follow any recent loss, injury, illness, or disenfranchisement.

202. Which of the following statements about grief is *false?*

a. Acute grief is an existential response that sooner or later normalizes.
b. Symptoms of acute grief include weeping, agitation, and helplessness.
c. Benzodiazepines are not indicated for sleep disturbances associated with acute grief.
d. Mourning is influenced by age, culture, community pressure, religious beliefs, and personal factors.
e. A primary mourner is the person who stands to lose the most by a recent death.

203. Which of the following statements about acute grief is *false?*

a. As a rule, statements made by well-meaning friends and family unwittingly attempt to abort the mourning process.
b. In general, sayings such as "Try to control yourself" are ineffective and counter-productive.
c. Death of a person or a relationship disapproved of by society may still lead to grief.
d. Frequently intervention depends on a balance between acceptance of a loss and denial of it.
e. Acute grief, in general, lasts for several weeks.

204. Which of the following statements about grief is *false?*

a. Acute and chronic losses precipitate grief.
b. The goal of the management of grief is to get rid of it as quickly as possible.
c. Listening is usually more effective than talking to those who are grief stricken.
d. Manifestations of acute grief tend to become less painful over time.
e. Clinicians should not force a grieving patient to talk about his or her loss.

205. Which of the following statements about pain is *false?*

a. Pain is one of the most common symptoms reported to physicians.
b. Pain is an unpleasant sensory and emotional experience arising from actual or potential tissue damage.
c. All pain has a psychological component.
d. Patients in pain often fear becoming addicted to analgesics.
e. Pain is usually diagnosed by use of objective tests.

206. Which of the following is *not* required for prescriptions of controlled substances, according to the Drug Enforcement Administration (DEA) guidelines?

a. Directions for use
b. Registration number of the practitioner
c. Home address of the patient
d. Telephone number of the practitioner
e. Address of the practitioner

207. Which of the following statements about pain is *false?*

a. Nociceptive pain results from direct tissue injury with or without damage to the nervous system.
b. Somatic nociceptive pain is usually attributed to certain anatomical structures.
c. Visceral pain is usually poorly localized.
d. Somatic pain is often described as aching or throbbing.
e. Visceral pain is often described as sharp, shooting, or burning pain.

For questions 208 to 211, match the terms in the left column with the definitions in the right column.

208. Allodynia
209. Hyperpathia
210. Hyperesthesia
211. Hyperalgesia

a. An increased response to stimuli that are normally painful
b. An exaggerated pain response to a noxious stimulus (e.g. heat)
c. Pain from a sensation not normally painful (e.g. light touch)
d. Pain from painful stimuli with delay and persistence beyond stimulation

212. Which of the following statements about reflex sympathetic dystrophy (RSD) is *false?*

a. RSD is a syndrome of pain in an extremity mediated by sympathetic overactivity that does not involve a major nerve.
b. RSD is a syndrome with sensory, autonomic, and motor features.
c. RSD is usually caused by a major injury.
d. Spontaneous pain occurs in a majority of cases of RSD.
e. Pain, edema, and warm skin may last up to six months with RSD.

213. Which of the following statements about sympathetically mediated pain is *false?*

a. It can be blocked by application of a local anesthetic to the sympathetic chain.
b. It can be blocked by application of intravenous phentolamine.
c. It can be blocked by application of intravenous guanethidine.
d. It can be blocked by application of serotonin agonists.
e. It can be blocked by application of spinal cord stimulation.

214. Which of the following is *not* a nonsteroidal anti-inflammatory drug?

a. Ibuprofen
b. Ketorolac
c. Terfenadine
d. Naproxen
e. Phenylbutazone

215. Which of the following narcotics listed below is *not* equipotent in analgesic effect to 10 mg of parenteral morphine sulfate?

a. Oral codeine 130 mg
b. Parenteral hydromorphone 1.5 mg
c. Parenteral meperidine 100 mg
d. Parenteral methadone 20 mg
e. Oral hydromorphone 7.5 mg

216. Which of the following author(s) is/are linked with the notion that there are seven distinct personality types seen among medical patients?

a. Elisabeth Kübler-Ross
b. Avery Weisman and Thomas Hackett
c. Ralph Kahana and Greta Bibring
d. Thomas Hackett and Ned Cassem
e. Flanders Dunbar

217. Which of the following personality types is not one of the seven types listed by the author(s) that described them?

a. Borderline
b. Dependent
c. Long-suffering
d. Guarded
e. Aloof

218. According to *DSM-IV* criteria, dementia includes an acquired deficit in memory and at least one other area of higher cortical function. Which of the following is *not* one of the areas on that list?

a. Agnosia
b. Aphasia
c. Aprosodia
d. Apraxia
e. Executive dysfunction (e.g., impairment of abstraction or planning)

For Questions 219 to 223, match the terms in the left column with the definitions in the right column.

219. Agnosia

220. Apraxia

221. Aphasia

222. Acalculia

223. Aprosodia

a. An inability to carry out motor tasks despite intact motor function

b. A failure to recognize familiar objects despite intact sensory function

c. A difficulty with language

d. An inability to interpret emotional cues or to convey them

e. An inability to calculate

224. Which of the following statements about dementia is *false?*

a. By age 85, the prevalence may be as high as 25%.

b. The prevalence in those over the age of 60 is 15%.

c. Homozygote apolipoprotein E4 alleles occur more commonly in patients with dementia of the Alzheimer's type than in those without it.

d. Dementia is associated with significant impairment in social or occupational function.

e. Not all dementias are progressive.

Questions 225 to 230 are *true-false* questions.

225. Dementia of the Alzheimer's type (DAT) has an insidious onset.

226. Dementia of the Alzheimer's type may be linked with a positive family history.

227. Pick's disease primarily affects the temporal lobes.

228. Creutzfeldt-Jakob disease is a rare, slowly progressive disorder caused by a prion.

229. Creutzfeldt-Jakob disease often is associated with myoclonus.

230. Tacrine and donepezil are each drugs that may provide transient benefit in cognition among patients with dementia of the Alzheimer's type; each requires monitoring of liver function tests.

For questions 231 to 235, match the brain regions in the left column with the behaviors listed in the right column.

231. Frontal	a. Dysgraphia
232. Parietal	b. Inappropriate behavior
233. Temporal	c. Confabulation
234. Thalamus	d. Aphasia
235. Striatum	e. Dysarthria

For questions 236 to 240, match the brain regions in the left column with the behaviors listed in the right column.

236. Frontal	a. Abulia
237. Parietal	b. Extrapyramidal movement disorder
238. Temporal	c. Sensory aprosodia
239. Thalamus	d. Confabulation
240. Striatum	e. Finger agnosia

For questions 241 to 245, match the signs in the left column with the associated conditions in the right column.

241. Butterfly rash	a. CHF
242. Café-au-lait spots	b. Systemic lupus erythematosus
243. Oral thrush	c. Encephalitis
244. Edema	d. Neurofibromatosis
245. Fever	e. HIV infection

Questions 246 to 250 are *true-false* questions.

246. Prosody, or the affective modulation of speech, is often impaired in patients with right hemispheric lesions.

247. Dysarthria is a pure motor dysfunction.

248. Hallucinations, commonly drug-induced, are misperceptions of sensory information in the real world.

249. Scores obtained on the Mini Mental State Examination (MMSE) should be adjusted according to the patient's age and educational level.

250. The Mini Mental State Examination (MMSE) is a good screening test for frontal lobe functioning.

For questions 251 to 255, match the type of aphasia in the left column with the manifestations of it in the right column.

251. Global
252. Wernicke's
253. Broca's
254. Conduction
255. Transcortical motor

a. Repetition impaired, comprehension intact, speech nonfluent
b. Repetition impaired, comprehension intact, speech fluent
c. Repetition impaired, comprehension impaired, speech nonfluent
d. Repetition intact, comprehension intact, speech nonfluent
e. Repetition impaired, comprehension impaired, speech fluent

For questions 256 to 260, match the terms in the left column with the definitions in the right column.

256. Dysnomia
257. Alexia
258. Abulia
259. Dyspraxia
260. Echopraxia

a. Involuntary imitation of movements made by another person
b. Difficulty executing purposeful movements, such as brushing the teeth
c. Lack of motivation to speak, move, or act
d. Word-finding difficulty
e. Inability to comprehend written material

For questions 261 to 265, match the terms in the left column with the definitions in the right column.

261. Hallucinations
262. Preoccupations
263. Hallucinosis
264. Illusions
265. Delusions

a. Perceptions of external stimuli that are misinterpreted
b. An ongoing series of hallucinatory experiences
c. Persistent and unshakable acceptances of false beliefs
d. Perceptions that occur in the absence of a corresponding sensory stimulus
e. Recurrences of thoughts that are neither unshakable nor necessarily false

266. Which type of hallucination is associated with the Charles Bonnet syndrome?

a. Visual
b. Auditory
c. Olfactory
d. Gustatory
e. Tactile

For questions 267 to 269, match the statements in the left column with the definitions in the right column.

267. Capgras syndrome
268. Delusions of de Fregoli
269. De Clerambault's syndrome

a. Where a person with erotomania believes he or she is having a relationship with an important, yet phantom lover
b. Where a person appears to change into many different people
c. Where a person believes a close relation is replaced by an impostor
d. Where a person believes he or she is infested with parasites
e. Where a person believes he or she has a Doppelganger (or self-double)

270. Which type of hallucinations are most common in schizophrenia?

a. Auditory
b. Olfactory
c. Tactile
d. Gustatory
e. Visual

271. Which type of hallucinations are most common in withdrawal states and drug intoxication?

a. Auditory
b. Olfactory
c. Tactile
d. Gustatory
e. Visual

272. Which of the following neuroleptics is *least* potent?

a. Chlorpromazine
b. Haloperidol
c. Thiothixene
d. Perphenazine
e. Molindone

273. Which of the following antipsychotics is the *most* anticholinergic?

a. Thiothixene
b. Clozapine
c. Risperidone
d. Perphenazine
e. Chlorpromazine

274. Approximately what percentage of the population will experience *at least* one seizure during their lifetime?

a. Less than five percent
b. Five to 10%
c. 10 to 15%
d. 15 to 20%
e. Greater than 20%

275. Which is the *most* common type of seizure?

a. Focal motor
b. Simple partial
c. Complex partial
d. Generalized
e. Petit mal

276. Roughly what percent of patients who have an unprovoked seizure will experience a second seizure?

a. Less than five percent
b. 15%
c. 30%
d. 45%
e. More than 60%

277. A seizure due to seizure activity limited to a single brain area is most likely a

a. Complex partial seizure
b. Simple partial seizure
c. Generalized seizure
d. Withdrawal seizure
e. Myoclonic seizure

278. Symptoms of a simple partial seizure include each of the following *except*

a. Motor phenomena
b. Sensory phenomena
c. Autonomic phenomena
d. Psychic phenomena
e. Alteration in consciousness

279. *True-false.* All complex partial seizures originate in the temporal lobe.

280. A seizure that spreads to closely connected areas and results in impaired consciousness is likely a

a. Complex partial seizure
b. Simple partial seizure
c. Generalized seizure
d. Withdrawal seizure
e. Myoclonic seizure

281. Precipitants of seizure include each of the following *except*

a. Alcohol
b. Fever
c. Sleep deprivation
d. Aerobic exercise
e. Incandescent lamps

282. *True-false.* Absence (petit mal) seizures are a type of generalized seizure.

283. Drugs commonly (i.e., greater than three percent of the time) associated with seizures include each of the following *except*

a. Maprotiline
b. Clozapine
c. Phencyclidine
d. Meperidine
e. Cyclosporine

284. *True-false.* An aura is a simple partial seizure with sensory or autonomic phenomena that may develop into a complex partial seizure with or without secondary generalization.

285. The first EEG obtained in patients with seizures shows epileptiform discharges (spikes or sharp waves) in roughly what percent of patients?

a. Less than 10%
b. 10%
c. 30%
d. 50%
e. More than 60%

Questions 286 to 289 are *true-false* questions.

286. Post-traumatic seizures typically occur more than one year after the injury.

287. The duration of a pseudo-seizure is typically longer than that of a seizure.

288. Post-ictal confusion or lethargy is often seen after a generalized seizure.

289. Thrashing, crying, pelvic thrusting, and a lack of self-injury are common with complex partial seizures.

290. Which of the following is a first-line anticonvulsant for absence seizures?

a. Phenytoin
b. Ethosuximide
c. Gabapentin
d. Phenobarbital
e. Carbamazepine

291. Which of the following anticonvulsants is a first-line treatment for partial seizures?

a. Lamotrigine
b. Carbamazepine
c. Gabapentin
d. Phenobarbital
e. Primidone

292. Therapeutic levels of 50 to 100 μg/mL are associated with use of which anticonvulsant?

a. Phenytoin
b. Carbamazepine
c. Valproic acid
d. Phenobarbital
e. Primidone

293. Therapeutic levels of 10 to 20 µg/mL are associated with use of which anticonvulsant?

a. Phenytoin
b. Carbamazepine
c. Valproic acid
d. Ethosuximide
e. Primidone

294. Which of the following statements about closed-head injuries is *false?*

a. Closed-head injuries result from nonpenetrating blows to the head with or without loss of consciousness.
b. A majority of symptoms experienced by patients in the initial phase post-concussion resolve by three to six months.
c. The primary brain injury in closed-head injury typically occurs in the anterior temporal lobes and the inferior surface of the frontal lobes.
d. Acceleration and deceleration forces may cause significant neuronal damage from sheer forces.
e. The yearly incidence of brain injury following concussive syndromes secondary to closed-head injury is roughly the same as in stroke.

295. Which of the following neurobehavioral symptoms is *not* typically a part of the post-concussive syndrome?

a. Dizziness
b. Perseveration
c. Mood lability
d. Hallucinations
e. Fatigue

296. Somatic manifestations of post-concussive syndrome include each of the following *except*

a. Diminished appetite
b. Headache
c. Sleep disturbance
d. Diminished libido
e. Dizziness

297. Affective symptoms of post-concussive syndrome include each of the following *except*

a. Irritability
b. Euphoria
c. Mood lability
d. Depression
e. Indifference

298. Cognitive symptoms associated with post-concussive syndrome include each of the following *except*

a. Diminished concentration
b. Diminished attention
c. Memory problems
d. Aphasia
e. Perseveration

299. Which of the following statements about cerebral concussion is *false?*

a. It may cause loss of consciousness.
b. It results in post-traumatic amnesia.
c. It may result in post-traumatic onset of seizures.
d. It rarely causes significant impairment in social or occupational function.
e. It is often associated with a normal EEG recording.

300. Which of the following statements about treatment strategies related to brain-injured patients is *false?*

a. Behavioral techniques help manage aggressive outbursts and inappropriate social behavior.
b. Vocational counseling and skills retraining may be helpful to work around deficits.
c. Family therapy and couples counseling may be helpful when dealing with personality changes following brain injury.
d. Brain-injured patients tolerate neuroleptics as well as do non-brain-injured patients.
e. Following closed-head injury, aggressive behavior may respond to antidepressants, buspirone, anticonvulsants, neuroleptics, and beta-blockers.

Questions 301 to 322 are *true-false* questions.

301. Computed tomography (CT) uses x-rays that are differentially attenuated depending on the material through which they pass.

302. Contrast media that enhances the visibility of pathology by CT are either ionic or nonionic.

303. Idiosyncratic reactions to contrast material occur in less than one percent of cases.

304. Ionic contrast material is more expensive than nonionic contrast material.

305. The risk of side-effects is roughly equivalent for ionic and nonionic contrast material.

306. Risk factors for contrast-induced side-effects include age less than 1 year or greater than 60 years.

307. Risk factors for contrast-induced side-effects include a history of asthma, allergies, cardiovascular disease, and prior contrast reactions.

308. CT offers spatial resolution of less than 1 mm.

309. CT scanning is useful for the detection of acute (i.e., less than 72 hours old) bleeding.

310. CT scanning is useful for the detection of bleeding in severely anemic patients (i.e., with a hemoglobin less than 10 g/dL).

311. CT is helpful in the visualization of subtle white matter lesions.

312. CT is not contraindicated in pregnancy.

313. Magnetic resonance imaging (MRI) exploits the magnetic properties of hydrogen atoms in water molecules.

314. T-1 weighted images are useful to detect areas of pathology.

315. Gadolinium causes fewer and less severe side-effects than does CT contrast material.

316. MRI scanning is superior to CT for visualization of white matter.

317. CT is superior to MRI or visualization of the posterior fossa and the brainstem.

318. Mechanical devices, such as pacemakers, can malfunction within the magnetic field of MRI scanners.

319. Positron emission tomography (PET) scanning measures cerebral blood flow.

320. PET scanning measures cerebral glucose metabolism.

321. PET scanning offers spatial resolution of less than 3 mm.

322. Single photon emission computed tomography (SPECT) provides better spatial resolution than PET scanning.

323. Which of the following is *not* typically an indication for CT imaging?
a. Dementia
b. New-onset psychosis
c. Movement disorder
d. Anorexia nervosa
e. Panic disorder

324. *True-false.* Rates for depression among amputees exceed those for victims of stroke.

325. Which of the following questions of the patient engaging in rehabilitation from a physical injury is *least* helpful?

a. What is the meaning of the injury or illness to the patient?
b. How does the patient's situation or condition affect self-image?
c. What is the patient's native language if he or she speaks more than one?
d. What does the patient think the effect of his or her situation is on family or friends?
e. How does the patient feel about his or her change or loss of function (e.g., work, sex, academic function)?

326. Which of the following statements about sexual function and dysfunction is *false?*

a. Roughly one-half of American couples suffer from some type of sexual problem.
b. Roughly one-fourth of Americans will experience a sexual dysfunction at some time in their lives.
c. Roughly five percent of medical outpatients present to their PCP with a sexual complaint.
d. The incidence of sexual problems in any medical practice is directly related to the frequency with which the clinician takes a sexual history.
e. Sexual dysfunction is best understood by having knowledge of the stages of abnormal sexual response.

327. *True-false.* The refractory period associated with normal sexual responses lengthens as the age of men and women increases.

328. Which of the following drugs is *least* likely to cause a reduction in libido?

a. Methyldopa
b. Thiazide diuretics
c. Thioridazine
d. Propranolol
e. Fluoxetine

329. *True-false. Dyspareunia* is the term used for a condition with persistent genital pain before, during, or after sexual intercourse in either the male or female.

330. Which of the following statements about premature ejaculation is *false?*

a. Premature ejaculation occurs in less than two minutes with less than 10 thrusts.
b. Premature ejaculation is the most common male sexual disorder; it occurs in 15% of men.
c. Prolonged periods without sexual activity often make the problem worse.
d. If the problem is chronic and untreated, secondary impotence often develops.
e. Premature ejaculation occurs with minimal stimulation before or after penetration and before the person wishes it.

331. Which of the following statements about impotence is *false?*

a. The frequency of erectile dysfunction increases as men get older.
b. By age 65, roughly 30% of men have erectile dysfunction.
c. Between five and 10% of men of all ages experience erectile dysfunction on a regular basis.
d. Impotence is one of the most common problems affecting men.
e. Aging by itself is not a cause of erectile dysfunction.

Questions 332 to 335 are *true-false* questions.

332. At least 50% of cases of erectile dysfunction have an organic basis.

333. The absence of nocturnal penile tumescence (NPT) suggests an organic disease.

334. Nocturnal penile tumescence occurs approximately every 90 minutes during non-REM sleep.

335. Erectile dysfunction is another name for Peyronie's disease.

336. Organically-based erectile dysfunction can be treated successfully with each of the following *except*

a. Clonidine
b. Yohimbine
c. Alprostadil
d. Papaverine
e. Testosterone

Questions 337 to 344 are *true-false* questions.

337. Infertility is defined as failure to conceive after three months of regular sexual intercourse or inability to carry a pregnancy to live birth.

338. Infertility is diagnosed in approximately 1 of every 12 couples of child-bearing age.

339. Roughly 25% of women under 25 years of age suffer from infertility.

340. Roughly 50% of women between 35 and 40 years of age suffer from infertility.

341. Roughly 25% of infertile patients report that the stress associated with infertility adversely affects their occupation and social function.

342. Sexual dysfunction occurs in up to one-half of women who receive treatment for infertility.

343. More than 50% of women suffer an episode of major depression during the first six months after a spontaneous abortion.

344. There is an increased rate of separation and divorce among couples who experience a pregnancy loss.

345. Which of the following statements is *not* part of the diagnostic criteria for premenstrual dysphoric disorder?
a. Marked affective lability
b. Marked anxiety or tension
c. Sleep disturbance
d. Brief psychotic episodes
e. Marked interference with work or school activities

Questions 346 to 347 are *true-false* questions.

346. Less than half of women with premenstrual dysphoric disorder have mood or anxiety disorders.

347. For menopause to be diagnosed, menses must be absent for 6 consecutive months.

348. The median age of the onset of the perimenopause, defined as the time of transition from regular menstrual function to the complete cessation of menses, is approximately

a. 42 years
b. 47 years
c. 52 years
d. 57 years
e. 62 years

349. *True-false.* The post-menopausal phase refers to the period after 12 months of amenorrhea, excluding cases of anorexia nervosa.

350. Risk factors that may predispose a patient to perimenopausal and menopausal mood disorders include each of the following *except*

a. A history of depression
b. A history of premenstrual syndrome
c. A history of premature menopause
d. A history of panic disorder
e. A history of post-partum depression

Questions 351 to 383 are *true-false* questions.

351. Hormone replacement therapy with estrogen is the cornerstone of the treatment of menopausal patients who present with physical, somatic, or cognitive complaints.

352. Hormone replacement therapy places some menopausal women at increased risk for breast and uterine cancer.

353. Estrogen monotherapy is an effective treatment for the depression that accompanies menopause.

354. The prevalence of major and minor depression during pregnancy is approximately five percent.

355. The strongest predictor of post-partum depression is affective disturbance during pregnancy.

356. When the frequency of congenital malformation after prenatal exposure to a medication is increased compared with the baseline incidence of congenital malformations without such drug exposure, the drug is labeled a teratogen.

357. Untreated major depression has been associated with a higher rate of neonatal complications and a lower Apgar score.

358. Low-potency antipsychotics are associated with increased risk of congenital malformations after first trimester exposure to these agents.

359. Extrapyramidal symptoms are rare in newborns born to mothers treated with neuroleptics during pregnancy.

360. Prenatal exposure to tricyclic antidepressants is not associated with an increased risk of organ dysgenesis after first trimester exposure.

361. Fluoxetine is not associated with an increased risk of congenital malformations after first trimester exposure.

362. Prenatal exposure to lithium carbonate during the first 12 weeks of gestation is associated with a risk for Goldstein's anomaly.

363. Although the risk for congenital malformations of the heart following lithium exposure during the first trimester is 10 times that of the risk for non-lithium-treated pregnant patients, the frequency of cardiac malformations is still relatively small.

364. Fewer than half of women with bipolar disorder relapse within the acute post-partum period.

365. Prophylaxis with mood stabilizers reduces the relapse rate of bipolar women to less than 10% post-partum.

366. Use of valproic acid is associated with less than a two to three percent risk of neural tube defects following first trimester exposure.

367. The risk for congenital malformations after first trimester exposure to valproic acid is 100 times the risk in lithium-treated pregnant women.

368. The risk for spina bifida after first trimester prenatal exposure to carbamazepine is three to five percent.

369. Post-partum blues is a time-limited condition involving mood lability that occurs in approximately 25 to 50% of post-partum women.

370. While post-partum blues is considered to be a normal reaction after childbirth, it may predict the risk for post-partum depression.

371. Symptoms of post-partum blues develop within two to three days of delivery and last up to six weeks.

372. Post-partum depression is defined as major depression that develops within one to two months of delivery.

373. Post-partum psychosis is a rare condition that occurs in 1 to 2 of every 1000 post-partum women.

374. The majority of women with post-partum psychosis are eventually diagnosed as having schizophrenia.

375. The majority of women with a history of major depression or bipolar disorder will develop a post-partum mood disorder.

376. Women with a history of post-partum psychosis have greater than a 90% risk for recurrent post-partum psychosis.

377. Post-partum thyroiditis is a risk factor for post-partum mood disorders.

378. Post-partum depression is time-limited, and for the majority of women with this condition reassurance is sufficient.

379. All psychotropics will be passed into the mother's breast milk.

380. Breast-feeding while the mother is taking lithium is not recommended.

381. According to *DSM-IV*, a traumatic event may involve witnessing a traumatic occurrence.

382. Traumatic events may lead to perceptual distortions of time, so that time may be slowed or accelerated.

383. Chronic exposure to trauma, or trauma that occurs in childhood, can produce long-lasting personality disturbances.

384. Which of the following statements about traumatic memories is *false?*
a. They have an intrusive quality.
b. They may intrude as nightmares.
c. They may lead to psychosis.
d. They are triggered by environmental cues that are associated with the traumatic event.
e. They may be associated with physiological arousal.

Questions 385 to 388 are *true-false* questions.

385. According to *DSM-IV,* an acute stress disorder is diagnosed when the response to trauma causes clinically significant impairment that lasts at least two weeks and occurs within four weeks of the traumatic experience.

386. According to *DSM-IV,* post-traumatic stress disorder is diagnosed when the characteristic trauma response causes clinically significant impairment lasting more than one month.

387. The lifetime risk for developing post-traumatic stress disorder in community samples is less than one percent.

388. More than 25% of rape victims experience post-traumatic stress disorder.

389. Evaluation of the person immediately following a traumatic event should include each of the following principles *except*
a. Establish rapport with the patient
b. Gently encourage the patient to review the trauma and surrounding events
c. Prepare the patient for the chronicity of the reactions to the trauma
d. Identify the aspect of the trauma that was most distressing to the patient
e. Pay attention to practical and immediate concerns brought on by the trauma

390. Treatment immediately following a traumatic event includes each of the following principles *except*
a. Convey whatever is known about the traumatic event to the patient
b. Educate the patient about the common responses to trauma
c. Use benzodiazepines liberally to decrease anxiety and sedate the patient
d. Review how the patient has previously managed crises to recall the patient's strengths
e. Encourage the patient to use existing supports

391. Which of the following statements about rape is *false?*
a. The legal definition of rape varies by state.
b. Criteria for rape include lack of consent, use of threat or force, and nonconsensual contact involving the breasts, genitals, or anus.
c. The prevalence of rape is increasing.
d. Date rape is a criminal act.
e. Hospital providers are in general mandated reporters of sexual assaults.

392. *True-false.* Male sexual assault victims generally do not seek medical or legal help.

393. Which of the following statements about the clinician's approach to the rape victim is *false?*

a. The majority of rape victims are evaluated in emergency rooms.
b. Rape victims in the emergency room want reassurance regarding their physical safety.
c. A measure of autonomy and control can be provided to a rape victim by explaining what to expect during the collection of evidence and during the physical exam.
d. Given the patient's emotional state in the emergency room, the clinician should guide the patient toward the decision to press charges against the assailant.
e. It is helpful to have the patient identify his or her needs and mobilize support systems.

394. Documentation of a sexual assault includes each of the following *except*

a. Documentation of the physical and emotional trauma related to the assault
b. Direct quotations from the patient
c. A detailed description of the assailant
d. A concise description of the event
e. Use of the term *reported* rather than *alleged*

Questions 395 to 399 are *true-false* questions.

395. Psychological reactions in the period immediately after a rape involve self-blame, fear of being killed, and recurrent intrusive thoughts.

396. When documenting the psychological responses of the patient, one should be comprehensive.

397. Unless a psychiatric disturbance is diagnosed by history or examination, inferences about psychiatric diagnoses should be avoided in the emergency room record of the rape victim.

398. Informed consent for treatment is not required for treatment of the rape victim.

399. Post-coital contraception is offered to the rape victim after a detailed menstrual history is taken and after the patient is advised about the options.

400. Which of the following statements about obsessive-compulsive disorder (OCD) is *false?*

a. One of the most common obsessions is a fear of contamination.
b. The lifetime prevalence of OCD is between two and three percent.
c. OCD commonly co-exists with other psychiatric disorders.
d. Because the symptoms of OCD are distressing, patients typically report their symptoms to their physicians.
e. Common compulsions include repetitive hand washing, checking, and counting.

Questions 401 to 406 are *true-false* questions.

401. Hoarding newspapers, spoiled food, wrappers, coupons, or useless clothes are common compulsions for those afflicted with OCD.

402. Body dysmorphic disorder (BDD) is a condition involving physical deformities that results in referrals for cosmetic surgery.

403. Tics are more common in patients with OCD than they are in the general population.

404. One-fourth to one-half of patients with OCD have obsessive-compulsive personality disorder (OCPD).

405. Patients with obsessive-compulsive personality disorder (OCPD) do not have obsessions or compulsions. Instead they have a lifelong pattern of over-attention to detail.

406. Which of the following medications is *least* effective for OCD?

a. Fluvoxamine
b. Fluoxetine
c. Clomipramine
d. Imipramine
e. Paroxetine

407. *True-false.* It is more common for a patient with OCD to have a partial remission of symptoms than a total remission with pharmacological treatment.

408. The lifetime prevalence of bipolar disorder is
a. Less than one percent
b. One to four percent
c. Five to eight percent
d. Nine to 12%
e. Greater than 12%

409. At any point in time, what percentage of those diagnosed with bipolar disorder are receiving medical treatment?
a. Less than 10%
b. 15 to 20%
c. 25 to 30%
d. 35 to 40%
e. Greater than 50%

410. Approximately what percentage of patients with bipolar disorder die by suicide?
a. Less than five percent
b. Five to 15%
c. 15 to 25%
d. 25 to 35%
e. Greater than 35%

411. The median duration of manic episodes of bipolar disorder is
a. Five weeks
b. 10 weeks
c. 15 weeks
d. 20 weeks
e. 25 weeks

412. *True-false.* For patients with bipolar disorder, the duration of well intervals between episodes tends to shrink progressively over the first three to five episodes.

413. Causes of secondary mania include each of the following conditions *except*

a. Thyrotoxicosis
b. Multiple sclerosis
c. Hypercalcemia
d. HIV infection
e. Systemic lupus erythematosus

414. First-line pharmacological treatment of acute episodes of cyclical mood disorder includes

a. Propranolol
b. Clonidine
c. Phototherapy
d. Valproic acid
e. Verapamil

Questions 415 to 416 are *true-false* questions.

415. Carbamazepine levels drop after 8 to 12 weeks of treatment owing to enzyme induction.

416. Maintenance treatment for bipolar disorder should continue for at least six months after the first and any subsequent manic episode.

417. *DSM-IV* criteria for a manic episode include each of the following *except*

a. Grandiosity
b. A distinct period of abnormally and persistently elevated, expansive, or irritable mood lasting at least one week or any duration if hospitalization is necessary
c. A decreased need for sleep
d. Delusions of persecution
e. Racing thoughts

418. *True-false.* Mania induced by antidepressant medication should not count toward a diagnosis of bipolar I disorder.

419. Significant contraindications to lithium therapy include each of the following *except*

a. Renal impairment
b. Hepatic dysfunction
c. Myasthenia gravis
d. Pregnancy
e. Fluid and salt imbalance

420. Major drug interactions occur between each of the following drugs and lithium *except*

a. Thiazide diuretics
b. Nonsteroidal anti-inflammatory drugs
c. ACE inhibitors
d. Calcium channel blockers
e. H2 blockers

421. Common side-effects associated with lithium therapy include each of the following *except*

a. Tremor
b. Weight gain
c. Psoriasis
d. Headache
e. Polyuria

422. Prior to lithium therapy, laboratory tests often recommended include each of the following *except*

a. Complete blood count
b. Electrolytes
c. BUN and creatinine
d. Thyroid function tests
e. Liver function tests

423. Significant contraindications to the use of clonazepam therapy for bipolar disorder include each of the following *except*

a. Narrow angle glaucoma
b. Sedative-hypnotic abuse
c. Alcohol abuse
d. A history of angina
e. A history of dyscontrol syndrome

424. Common adverse effects of valproic acid include each of the following *except*

a. Tremor
b. Sedation
c. Psoriasis
d. Headache
e. Nausea

425. Worrisome adverse effects of carbamazepine therapy include each of the following *except*

a. Aplastic anemia
b. Thrombocytopenia
c. Hypernatremia
d. Toxic epidermal necrolysis
e. Hepatitis

426. *True-false.* Patients with eating disorders often do not obtain psychiatric treatment or delay for years before starting treatment.

427. Which of the following statements about anorexia nervosa is *false?*

a. Anorexia nervosa is a syndrome involving a disturbance in body image that leads to self-starvation.
b. Patients with anorexia nervosa see themselves as being too fat.
c. In post-menarchal females with anorexia nervosa, at least six consecutive menstrual cycles are absent.
d. Patients with anorexia nervosa suffer from a consuming fear of weight gain.
e. Patients with anorexia nervosa purge by use of laxatives, vomiting, or excessive exercise.

428. Which of the following statements about bulimia nervosa is *false?*

a. Bulimia nervosa is a syndrome characterized by frequent episodes of binge eating during which the patient eats large amounts of food and feels unable to control his or her food intake.
b. Weight fluctuations are common among patients with bulimia nervosa.
c. To prevent weight gain, patients with bulimia nervosa purge by vomiting, taking laxatives, or exercising excessively.
d. Approximately one-fourth of patients with anorexia nervosa have bulimia symptoms.
e. Bulimia nervosa commonly begins in normal-weight or overweight females who have tried various diets.

429. Approximately what percent of eating-disordered patients are male?

a. Less than two percent
b. Two to five percent
c. Five to 10%
d. 11 to 15%
e. Greater than 15%

Questions 430 to 431 are *true-false* questions.

430. A higher percent of adolescent and young adult women suffer from anorexia nervosa than do adult women with bulimia nervosa.

431. The mortality associated with anorexia is less than two percent.

432. Which of the following features or conditions is *least* likely to be associated with bulimia nervosa?

a. Parotidomegaly
b. Lanugo (fine hair on the face and arms)
c. Perimolysis (enamel loss)
d. Abrasions on the metacarpopharyngeal joints (Russell's sign)
e. Signs of dehydration

433. Which of the following features or conditions is the *least* likely to be associated with anorexia nervosa?

a. Lanugo
b. Bradycardia
c. Polycystic ovaries
d. Hypotension
e. Hypothermia

Questions 434 to 437 are *true-false* questions.

434. Congestive heart failure may develop in patients with anorexia nervosa on refeeding.

435. Osteoporosis is a complication of anorexia nervosa.

436. Bupropion, but not desipramine, has been associated with an increased risk of seizures in patients with bulimia.

437. Obesity is defined as 150% of ideal body weight and is characterized by excess adipose tissue.

438. Approximately what percent of adult Americans are obese?

a. Five to 15%
b. 15 to 25%
c. 25 to 35%
d. 35 to 45%
e. Greater than 45%

439. Obesity-associated conditions or complications include each of the following *except*

a. Coronary artery disease
b. Cerebrovascular accidents
c. Hypertension
d. Narcolepsy
e. Sleep apnea

440. Each of the following psychotropics is associated with weight gain *except*

a. Mirtazapine
b. Phenelzine
c. Bupropion
d. Lithium
e. Olanzapine

Questions 441 to 442 are *true-false* questions.

441. Testing the stool for phenolphthalein may help identify the patient who has Cushing's syndrome.

442. Mental retardation is associated with higher rates of obesity than are present in the general population.

443. Each of the following agents has been found effective in achieving weight loss *except*

a. Sibutramine
b. Dexfenfluramine
c. Phentermine
d. Phenylpropanolamine
e. Cyproheptadine

444. Criteria for Acquired Immune Deficiency Syndrome (AIDS) in HIV-positive patients include each of the following *except*

a. CD4 cell count less than 200
b. Percentage of total lymphocytes below 14
c. Kaposi's sarcoma
d. Hepatitis
e. Candidiasis of the esophagus

445. *True-false.* Major depression is one of the most frequent major psychiatric complications of HIV infection and AIDS.

446. Common CNS opportunistic infections in HIV-infected patients include each of the following *except*

a. Histoplasmosis
b. Toxoplasmosis
c. Cryptococcosis
d. Candidiasis
e. Mycobacterium avium intracellulare

447. *True-false.* The presence of systemic HIV disease and HIV-associated CNS infection increases the risk of side-effects from conventional psychiatric medications.

448. Zidovudine (AZT) is associated with each of the following *except*

a. Headache
b. Peripheral neuropathy
c. Agitation
d. Insomnia
e. Mania

449. Acyclovir is associated with each of the following *except*

a. Loss of appetite
b. Visual hallucinations
c. Confusion
d. Hyperacusis
e. Insomnia

450. Which of the following is associated with pentamidine treatment?

a. Hypoglycemia
b. Euphoria
c. Visual hallucinations
d. Insomnia
e. Hyperacusis

Questions 451 to 457 are *true-false* questions.

451. HIV infects the brain early in the course of infection, but the frequency and severity of clinically important HIV CNS infections generally parallel those of systemic HIV disease.

452. HIV-associated dementia affects only five percent of patients with otherwise asymptomatic HIV infection.

453. Use of psychostimulants (e.g., dextroamphetamine and methylphenidate) may reduce the symptoms of decreased attention and concentration as well as apathetic mood in those with HIV infection.

454. Painful peripheral neuropathies commonly result from HIV infection and the neurotoxic side effects of nucleoside anti-retroviral agents.

455. Patients with HIV infection or AIDS are at no higher risk of suicide than are those with other chronic diseases like diabetes.

456. An HLA identical match takes precedence in the assignment of a cadaveric kidney.

457. Psychiatric exclusion criteria for transplantation differ among transplant centers.

458. Which of the following statements about noncompliance is *false* regarding patients undergoing organ transplantation?
a. Noncompliance is difficult to predict.
b. Noncompliance may present as missed medication, missed appointments, or failure to make a timely report of important symptomatic changes.
c. Noncompliance is not a reason to exclude a patient from a transplant list.
d. Great distances from a transplant center may increase the chance for noncompliance.
e. Assessment of noncompliance involves knowledge of cognitive deficits, presence of depression, and prior noncompliance.

459. Which of the following objectives of psychiatric screening of potential recipients of organs is *not* a priority?

a. To define a patient's belief about, and motivation for, transplantation
b. To identify preoperative psychiatric syndromes
c. To define the availability of social supports
d. To educate the patient about surgical risks and benefits
e. To advocate for the patient's moving up on a transplant list because of his or her social status

460. Contraindications to transplantation include each of the following *except*

a. Active suicidal ideation
b. Dementia
c. Active substance abuse
d. A history of substance abuse
e. Intractable noncompliance

461. *True-false.* SSRIs are well tolerated in patients with end-organ failure.

462. Which of the following statements about homelessness is *false?*

a. Single adults make up the majority of the homeless.
b. Veterans, whether combat exposed or not, make up 30 to 40% of homeless men.
c. Ethnic minorities are over-represented among the homeless.
d. A person who sleeps transiently in a series of friends' apartments meets a definition for homelessness.
e. Homelessness is synonymous with mental illness.

463. *True-false.* The majority of homeless adults report having one or no confidants, one or no friends, or one or no family members with whom they are in contact.

464. Schizophrenia is diagnosed in homeless adults roughly how much more often than in individuals with regular housing?

a. Less than 5 times
b. 15 to 25 times
c. 25 to 35 times
d. 35 to 45 times
e. Greater than 50 times

465. Alcohol abuse is present in roughly what percent of homeless adults?

a. Less than 15%
b. 15 to 30%
c. 30 to 45%
d. 45 to 60%
e. Greater than 60%

466. *True-false.* Chronic lung disease associated with smoking is more than 10 times more common in the homeless than it is in a matched housed sample.

467. Approximately what percent of homeless adults report having had psychiatric hospitalizations?

a. Less than 15%
b. 15 to 30%
c. 30 to 45%
d. 45 to 60%
e. Greater than 60%

468. Noncompliance with medical appointments for homeless adults is *least* likely related to which of the following statements?

a. Attendance at an appointment may mean giving up a basic necessity, such as food or a bed.
b. Appointment slips are often lost.
c. Memory disturbance may mean not keeping appointments on time.
d. Phone call or postal card reminders are frequently impossible.
e. Homeless patients may be made to feel uncomfortable by their clinicians.

Questions 469 to 471 are *true-false* questions.

469. Skin lesions in the homeless may be exacerbated by reaching into trash bins for recyclables.

470. Loud snoring characteristic of obstructive sleep apnea may cause ejection of a homeless patient from a shelter.

471. Since most homeless patients lead lives exposed to public view, confidentiality in the medical setting is not crucial.

472. In addition to the usual historical information, special attention should be paid to each of the following in the homeless *except*

a. Trauma
b. Sexually transmitted disease
c. Vaccinations
d. PPD test results
e. Renal function

Questions 473–476 are *true-false* questions.

473. The inconvenience of multiple dosing schedules makes once-daily dosing preferable among homeless adults.

474. In general, difficulty in treating celebrities occurs not because they are entitled, demanding, or seductive but because of the publicity that surrounds them.

475. Treating a celebrity enables a clinician to vicariously taste power.

476. Celebrities by definition have narcissistic personality disorder.

477. According to *DSM-IV,* criteria for narcissistic personality disorder include each of the following *except*

a. A lust for power through beauty, love, brilliance, or money
b. Entitlement
c. Success in business
d. Stunted empathy
e. Displays of contempt

Questions 478 to 498 are *true-false* questions.

478. Family members of celebrities may expect to be treated as demi-celebrities.

479. The physician who treats a celebrity patient should keep all members of the celebrity's coterie fully informed about medical events and progress.

480. In the medical setting, the use of an alias by a celebrity patient is often wise.

481. The physician caring for a celebrity patient should not become excited, fantasize, or wish for power.

482. The physician who treats a physician need not explain the illness or ongoing treatment to the patient, as he or she is likely to be familiar with it.

483. Issues related to substance abuse in the VIP should be avoided because of fears that the media will attempt to gather and use such information.

484. When conducting a family crisis meeting, each family member should be given the opportunity to explain without interruption and qualifications from others his or her unique perspective of the problem.

485. Providing a context of safety and comfort during a family crisis meeting is not essential.

486. During a family crisis meeting, the identified patient's problem is the focus of the meeting.

487. During a family crisis meeting, it helps to show an appreciation for the interests of all the family's concerns or distress about its difficulty.

488. During a family crisis meeting, redefining a problem in a way that points to a new direction of action is often helpful.

489. Family therapy is not contraindicated when one family member is violent.

490. Family therapy is a substitute for other therapies.

491. Less than one-fourth of all marriages involve physical violence at some point.

492. More than one-third of homicides occur within the family.

493. Women are injured or killed by domestic violence far more frequently than are men.

494. Abused women develop physical symptoms, depression, anxiety, somatic complaints, and substance abuse as often as do nonabused women.

495. Batterers are a demographically heterogeneous group.

496. A large percent of violent men abuse drugs or alcohol.

497. Abusive men often appear more believable than their abused partners.

498. The male batterer often is pathologically jealous of his female partner and accuses her of sexual infidelity.

499. Which of the following statements is *least* likely to account for women staying in violent relationships?
a. A battered woman may be trapped economically.
b. A battered woman may blame herself.
c. A battered woman may consider violence the price of a relationship with the abuser.
d. A battered woman may be rebelling against her own parents' wishes.
e. A battered woman may be too frightened to leave.

Questions 500 to 501 are *true-false* questions.

500. Patients rarely volunteer information about abuse spontaneously.

501. Multiple visits to an emergency room for any reason should raise concern that the patient is being abused.

502. The prevalence of psychosocial difficulty in all children is approximately what percent?

a. Less than five percent
b. Five to 10%
c. 10 to 15%
d. 15 to 20%
e. Greater than 20%

503. *True-false.* Children with difficulties in one area of functioning rarely demonstrate symptoms or difficulties in other areas of their daily functioning.

504. Which of the following areas is *least* useful to assess in children?

a. Cognitive status
b. Temperament
c. Ability to play team sports
d. Sociability
e. Family relations

505. Which of the following statements about attention deficit hyperactivity disorder (ADHD) is true?

a. Symptoms must be associated with impairment in school.
b. Symptoms must have begun before age 10 to qualify for the diagnosis.
c. Hyperactivity must be manifested by impatience.
d. The essential feature is a persistent pattern of inattention, hyperactivity, and impulsivity that is more frequent and severe than is typically observed in individuals of comparable levels of development.
e. The prevalence in children is estimated at two percent.

Questions 506 to 508 are *true-false* questions.

506. It is uncommon for ADHD to persist into adulthood.

507. ADHD is more prevalent in males than females.

508. Because of patient confidentiality, history about the symptoms of ADHD should be obtained from the patient and not from teachers.

509. Approximately what percentage of children with ADHD suffer from learning disabilities?

a. Less than 10%
b. 10 to 15%
c. 15 to 20%
d. 20 to 25%
e. Greater than 25%

510. *True-false.* Pemoline is longer-acting than is methylphenidate.

511. The typical starting dose for pemoline in children with ADHD is

a. 2.5 to 5 mg
b. 5 to 10 mg
c. 7.5 to 15 mg
d. 18.75 to 37.5 mg
e. 50 mg

512. The typical starting dose of methylphenidate in children with ADHD is

a. 2.5 to 5 mg
b. 5 to 10 mg
c. 7.5 to 15 mg
d. 18.75 to 37.5 mg
e. 50 mg

513. *True-false.* Concomitant use of stimulants and tricyclic antidepressants does not lead to changes in the serum level of the medications.

514. Which of the following drugs is *least* likely to be helpful to children with ADHD?

a. Pemoline
b. Desipramine
c. Clonidine
d. Verapamil
e. Selegiline

515. Complications of cocaine abuse and dependence involve each of the following *except*

a. Anosmia
b. Acute myocardial infarction
c. Stroke
d. Nasal polyps
e. Pulmonary edema

516. Complications of cocaine abuse and dependence include each of the following *except*

a. Seizures
b. Arrhythmias
c. Nephrolithiasis
d. Perforation of the nasal septum
e. Hepatitis

Questions 517 to 518 are *true-false* questions.

517. Cocaine metabolites may be detected in the urine for a longer time than metabolites of amphetamine.

518. Metabolites of cannabinoids can be detected in the urine more than three weeks after use of marijuana.

519. According to the *DSM-IV,* criteria for substance dependence include each of the following *except*

a. The development of tolerance
b. A persistent desire to use or unsuccessful efforts to cut down
c. Excessive time spent obtaining, using, or recovering from a substance
d. Continued use despite knowledge of problems
e. Seizures on withdrawal of the drug

520. Pharmacologic management of cocaine craving and withdrawal may include use of each of the following *except*

a.   Bromocriptine
b.   Desipramine
c.   Amantadine
d.   Mazindol
e.   Labetalol

521. Signs and symptoms of opiate withdrawal typically include each of the following *except*

a.   Yawning
b.   Lacrimation
c.   Decreased respiratory rate
d.   Rhinorrhea
e.   Dilated pupils

522. The lifetime prevalence of alcohol dependence among cocaine-dependent individuals is approximately what percentage?

a.   Less than 15%
b.   15 to 30%
c.   30 to 45%
d.   45 to 60%
e.   Greater than 60%

523. Life-threatening causes of agitation include each of the following *except*

a.   Hypoglycemia
b.   Hypertension
c.   Intracranial bleeding
d.   Meningitis
e.   Normal-pressure hydrocephalus

524. Life-threatening causes of agitation include each of the following *except*

a.   Hypoxia
b.   General paresis
c.   Poisoning
d.   Wernicke's encephalopathy
e.   Withdrawal from barbiturates

525. Heralds of impending violence typically include each of the following *except*

a.   Loud, fast speech
b.   Increased muscle tension
c.   Pacing
d.   Staring
e.   Talking to oneself

526. When interviewing and examining a violent or potentially violent patient, useful strategies include each of the following *except*

a.   Accepting what the patient tells you
b.   Expressing concern for the patient
c.   Attending to the patient's physical comfort
d.   Agreeing to whatever the patient asks for to avoid a crisis
e.   Using calm, nonthreatening language

527. When interviewing and examining a violent or potentially violent patient, useful strategies include each of the following *except*

a.   Avoiding continuous unbroken eye contact
b.   Gently touching the patient whenever possible
c.   Not crowding the patient
d.   Moving slowly and deliberately
e.   Maintaining a relaxed posture

528. The best predictor of violence or dangerous behavior is

a.   Numerous tattoos
b.   A prior history of violence or dangerous behavior
c.   Use of profane speech
d.   A history of suicide attempts
e.   A history of cocaine abuse

Questions 529 to 531 are *true-false* questions.

529. Violence is more likely to occur when a thought disorder is present.

530. When interviewing the potentially violent patient, it is best to be nonthreatening and to interview the patient alone so as not to threaten the patient by the presence of security personnel.

531. Alcohol intoxication is a common cause of violence in patients brought to emergency rooms.

532. Pharmacologic agents *least* likely to be used in the chronic management of aggressive behavior include

a. Neuroleptics
b. Antidepressants
c. Anticonvulsants
d. Lithium
e. Beta-blockers

533. Common indications for use of glucocorticoids include each of the following *except*

a. Bronchial asthma
b. Acute tubular necrosis
c. Multiple sclerosis
d. Spinal cord injuries
e. Systemic lupus erythematosus

For questions 534 to 538, match the name of the glucocorticoid preparation in the left column with the appropriate dose equivalent in the right column.

534. Prednisone a. 4 mg
535. Methylprednisolone b. 5 mg
536. Dexamethasone c. 25 mg
537. Cortisone d. 0.75 mg
538. Hydrocortisone e. 20 mg

539. Adverse effects of glucocorticoids include each of the following *except*

a. Thin, fragile skin
b. Osteoporosis
c. Myopathy
d. Peptic ulcers
e. Acute tubular necrosis

540. *True-false.* Affective symptoms are more common than psychosis and delirium after steroid use.

541. Neuropsychiatric effects of glucocorticoid use commonly include each of following *except*

a. Delirium
b. Depression
c. Mild euphoria
d. Panic attacks
e. Mania

542. Which of the following statements about glucocorticoid treatments is *false?*

a. Up to 30% of glucocorticoid-treated patients develop at least mild psychiatric symptoms.
b. Roughly five percent of glucocorticoid-treated patients develop severe psychiatric syndromes including depression, mania, psychosis, and delirium.
c. Neuropsychiatric symptoms generally start after several months of ongoing glucocorticoid treatment.
d. Among the patients who develop psychiatric complications secondary to glucocorticoid treatment, roughly 40% develop symptoms in the first week of treatment.
e. Most patients recover from their psychiatric symptoms within six weeks of discontinuation of glucocorticoids.

Questions 543 to 548 are *true-false* questions.

543. Women are more likely than are men to develop psychiatric sequelae from glucocorticoid use.

544. A history of psychiatric illness is a clear risk factor for the development of psychiatric symptoms from glucocorticoids.

545. The presence of a psychiatric syndrome during a prior course of glucocorticoid treatment predicts the reaction to a future course of treatment.

546. Only certain steroid preparations produce neuropsychiatric side-effects.

547. Neuropsychiatric symptoms similar in nature to those associated with use of glucocorticoids develop in patients with SLE in the absence of steroid treatment.

548. Approximately one percent of patients receiving less than 40 mg per day of prednisone will develop neuropsychiatric symptoms.

549. Approximately what percent of patients receiving more than 80 mg per day of prednisone will develop neuropsychiatric side-effects?

a. Less than one percent
b. One to five percent
c. Five to 15%
d. 15 to 25%
e. Greater than 50%

550. Symptoms associated with steroid withdrawal include each of the following *except*

a. Depression
b. Fatigue
c. Anxiety
d. Confusion
e. Seizures

551. Which of the following is *not* usually part of the management of patients receiving psychotropics?

a. Exploring the meaning of medication to the patient
b. Exploring the meaning of the diagnosis to the patient
c. Education of both the patient and the family regarding diagnosis and treatment
d. Treatment of target symptoms
e. Negotiating with pharmacies about unit pricing of medication

552. Which of the following is *not* true about compliance related to medication use?

a. QD dosing schedules enhance compliance.
b. If more than one medication is being taken, having the patient take medications at the same time enhances compliance.
c. It may be useful to acknowledge the difficulty of taking medication daily.
d. Monitoring of blood levels of selected medications may facilitate proper use of medication.
e. Roughly 25% of patients alter the way they take their medications.

553. Which of the following *most* often causes orthostatic hypotension?

a. Nortriptyline
b. Phenelzine
c. Fluoxetine
d. Bupropion
e. Mirtazapine

554. Which of the following *least* often causes orthostatic hypotension?

a. Nortriptyline
b. Phenelzine
c. Tranylcypromine
d. Bupropion
e. Trazodone

555. Which of the following *most* often causes prolongation of the QRS interval?

a. Imipramine
b. Phenelzine
c. Fluoxetine
d. Trazodone
e. Bupropion

556. Which of the following is *most* anticholinergic?

a. Desipramine
b. Clomipramine
c. Phenelzine
d. Paroxetine
e. Trazodone

557. Which of the following is the *least* sedating?

a. Trazodone
b. Bupropion
c. Clomipramine
d. Doxepin
e. Mirtazapine

558. Which of the following is the *most* sedating?

a. Trazodone
b. Bupropion
c. Protriptyline
d. Tranylcypromine
e. Desipramine

559. Which of the following is *most* likely to be associated with weight gain?

a. Phenelzine
b. Fluoxetine
c. Fluvoxamine
d. Bupropion
e. Trazodone

560. Which of the following is *least* likely to cause sexual dysfunction?

a. Clomipramine
b. Bupropion
c. Phenelzine
d. Paroxetine
e. Sertraline

Questions 561 to 562 are *true-false* questions.

561. Orthostatic hypotension is more common with MAOIs than with SSRIs.

562. Among the TCAs, nortriptyline has the lowest propensity to induce hypotension.

563. Treatment of an MAOI-induced hypotensive crisis may involve use of

a. Alpha methyldopa
b. Metaraminol
c. Isoproterenol
d. Nifedipine
e. Tramadol

564. Which of the following is *least* likely to create a risk of hypertensive crisis in a patient taking an MAOI?

a. Cottage cheese
b. Red wine
c. Soy sauce
d. Cured meats
e. Broad bean pods

565. Which of the following is the *most* likely to create a risk of hypertensive crisis in a patient taking an MAOI?

a. Aged cheese
b. Red wine
c. Chocolate
d. Bananas
e. Avocados

566. Sinus tachycardia is *most* likely in patients taking which of the following?

a. Clomipramine
b. Trazodone
c. Venlafaxine
d. Bupropion
e. Fluoxetine

567. H_2 blockers that treat nausea and dyspepsia include each of the following *except*

a. Ranitidine
b. Bethanechol
c. Cisapride
d. Metoclopramide
e. Famotidine

568. Treatments for diarrhea include each of the following *except*

a. Diphenoxylate
b. Bethanechol
c. Cyproheptadine
d. Lactobacillus acidophilus
e. Loperamide

569. MAOI-induced paresthesias may be treated by which of the following?

a. Trazodone
b. Pyridoxine
c. Cyproheptadine
d. Zolpidem
e. Amantadine

570. Anti-cholinergic effects of TCAs and SSRIs include each of the following *except*

a. Xerostomia
b. Blurred vision
c. Urinary retention
d. Decreased temperature
e. Memory loss

571. Priapism is *most* common with which of the following?

a. Yohimbine
b. Trazodone
c. Bupropion
d. Buspirone
e. Amantadine

572. Erectile and orgasmic dysfunction can be treated with each of the following *except*

a. Yohimbine
b. Trazodone
c. Amantadine
d. Bupropion
e. Cyproheptadine

Questions 573 to 635 are *true-false* questions.

573. All TCAs prolong the His-ventricular (H-V) interval and increase the risk of orthostatic hypotension in the presence of bundle branch block.

574. TCAs often decrease the frequency of premature ventricular contractions (PVCs).

575. Use of SSRIs may decrease the levels of beta-blockers.

576. Lithium levels remain stable when thiazide diuretics are administered.

577. Use of TCAs is often associated with bradyarrhythmia.

578. Use of lithium should be avoided in the presence of sick sinus syndrome.

579. TCAs should be avoided in the presence of first-degree AV block.

580. TCAs should be avoided in patients with prolonged QTc intervals.

581. Serum levels of carbamazepine may be raised by use of calcium channel blockers.

582. Serum levels of carbamazepine may be raised by use of erythromycin.

583. Droperidol causes less hypotension than does haloperidol.

584. Torsade des pointes is another name for hyperacute T waves.

585. Bupropion has a greater affinity for muscarinic anticholinergic receptors than does sertraline.

586. Venlafaxine has a greater affinity for muscarinic anticholinergic receptors than does sertraline.

587. Paroxetine has a greater affinity for muscarinic anticholinergic receptors than does fluoxetine.

588. QTc intervals greater than 440 milliseconds are considered to be abnormal.

589. When a QRS complex is greater than 100 milliseconds, it is termed a right bundle branch block.

590. Bupropion is not associated with serious cardiovascular toxicity.

591. Venlafaxine is chemically unrelated to other antidepressants.

592. Tertiary TCAs include amitriptyline, imipramine, and protriptyline.

593. Secondary TCAs include desipramine, nortriptyline, and trimipramine.

594. The risk of orthostatic hypotension associated with use of TCAs increases in patients with congestive heart failure.

595. Neuroleptic potency is a function of binding affinity for D_2 receptors in the CNS.

596. Thiothixene is more potent than perphenazine.

597. Trifluoperazine is equipotent to thiothixene.

598. Metoclopramide and promethazine each have neuroleptic properties.

599. Clozapine blocks D_2 receptors more than $5\text{-}HT_2$ receptors.

600. Up to 10% of clozapine-treated patients develop sinus tachycardia.

601. Risperidone acts primarily at $5\text{-}HT_2$ receptors rather than at D_2 receptors.

602. Risperidone, unlike clozapine, lacks muscarinic anticholinergic activity.

603. Quetiapine lacks muscarinic anticholinergic activity.

604. Lithium has little impact on the duration of the QRS complex.

605. Dextroamphetamine's half-life is longer than the half-life for methylphenidate.

606. Most drug-drug interactions involving psychotropic medications and nonpsychotropics do not contraindicate the combined use of those drugs.

607. Medications with a low therapeutic index achieve therapeutic levels quickly.

608. Lithium and warfarin are each drugs with a low therapeutic index.

609. Medications with a narrow therapeutic window are relatively ineffective above a specified therapeutic range.

610. Nortriptyline is a drug with a narrow therapeutic window.

611. Idiosyncratic reactions are rare but predictable reactions given knowledge of pharmacokinetics and pharmacodynamic properties.

612. Pharmacokinetic reactions involve interactions mediated by a direct effect on tissue receptor sites.

613. Absorption, distribution, metabolism, and excretion mediate pharmacokinetic interactions.

614. Metoclopramide slows gastric emptying.

615. Drug distribution from the systemic circulation to tissue is in part determined by regional blood flow.

616. Lithium is highly protein-bound.

617. Common inhibitors of hepatic metabolic enzymes include ketocona-zole, cimetidine, erythromycin, and phenytoin.

618. Inhibitors of hepatic metabolic enzymes typically produce an abrupt elevation in the blood levels of the co-administered drug.

619. Discontinuation of an inhibitor of hepatic metabolic enzymes is asso-ciated with a rapid fall in blood levels of a co-administered drug.

620. Inducers of hepatic metabolic enzymes produce an abrupt decline in the blood levels of the co-administered drug.

621. Inducers of the 3A3/4 P450 enzyme system include carbamazepine, phenobarbital, and phenytoin.

622. Addition of an ACE inhibitor to lithium decreases lithium levels.

623. Addition of theophylline to lithium increases lithium levels.

624. The co-administration of lithium and succinylcholine prolongs the duration of muscle paralysis.

625. The addition of carbamazepine to valproate raises valproate levels.

626. Lithium is more than 95% eliminated by the kidney.

627. The addition of carbamazepine to TCAs decreases TCA levels.

628. The addition of secondary amine TCAs to SSRIs raises TCA levels.

629. The addition of haloperidol to SSRIs raises the level of the neuroleptic.

630. The addition of propranolol to SSRIs lowers levels of beta-blockers.

631. Bupropion is *not* considered to be an inhibitor of the P450 isoen-zymes.

632. Mirtazapine is *not* considered to be an inhibitor of the P450 isoenzymes.

633. Trazodone is *not* considered to be an inhibitor of the P450 isoenzymes.

634. The addition of carbamazepine to neuroleptics lowers the level of the neuroleptic.

635. Addition of antacids delays the absorption of neuroleptics.

636. The goals of time-limited interviewing include each of the following *except*
a. Compilation of sufficient information to generate a differential diagnosis
b. Establishment of a relationship from which an effective treatment plan can be designed and implemented
c. Psychologizing about a medical psychiatric condition
d. Creation of an atmosphere in which the patient can convey information that may be shameful or frightening
e. Creation of a psychoeducational approach to define the problem and pave the way to a solution

637. When creating an atmosphere conducive to self-revelation, the clinician should consider each of the following *except*
a. Consider sharing what you already know about the problem or situation and invite correction.
b. Establish a mutual perspective.
c. Appreciate the patient's perspective.
d. Assume that the patient sees the problem the same way you do.
e. Get permission to discuss the problem before jumping in.

638. When getting data in a time-limited interview, strategies include each of the following *except*
a. Rely on a symptom checklist to rule a diagnosis out or in.
b. Let the patient tell his or her own story.
c. Explain what you are doing and why when moving to different features of the history.
d. Establish the last time the patient felt well with respect to the problem.
e. Summarize, reflect, and invite correction.

639. When approaching a sensitive subject in a time-limited interview, include each of the following *except*

a. Change the subject if you become anxious about your decision.
b. Be aware of the problem and plan for it.
c. Approach the problem indirectly at first.
d. Ask permission to bring up something that may be somewhat difficult to discuss.
e. Use open-ended questions to deepen the discussion.

640. Which of the following statements about cognitive-behavioral therapy (CBT) is *false?*

a. CBT is short-term, and the length of therapy is dependent on the time needed to help the patient develop alternative patterns of responses.
b. CBT is active and provides the patient with information.
c. CBT is unstructured and depends on the context of day-to-day events.
d. CBT is collaborative between the patient and the therapist.
e. CBT is focused on the modification of emotions and behavior.

641. *True-false.* In CBT, motivation is seen as a behavioral state that is modifiable and a focus of treatment.

642. Which of the following statements about CBT is *false?*

a. Information about symptoms that define a disorder helps reduce self-blame and/or catastrophic misinterpretations of symptoms.
b. Information about symptoms sets the stage for active collaboration between the clinician and the patient.
c. Information about the nature of the disorder enhances patient motivation for therapeutic change.
d. Treatment motivation and goal achievement are aided by clear specification and monitoring of goals and goal-directed activity by both the patient and the therapist.
e. Self-monitoring of symptoms is rarely part of the treatment plan in CBT.

643. Which of the following statements about exposure interventions in CBT is *false?*

a. Exposure is designed to allow maladaptive emotional responses to dissipate on continued successful exposure to a situation or event.
b. Exposure treatments may include direct exposure to feared situations.
c. Exposure can be conducted in a gradual stepwise fashion.
d. Exposure should terminate before anxiety starts to develop.
e. Exposure can be conducted as an extended exposure to strong cues.

Questions 644 to 649 are *true-false* questions.

644. CBT for social phobia usually emphasizes cognitive restructuring to alter anxiety-producing social expectations, and use of exposure to help patients develop skills and to decrease anxiety as part of social rehearsal.

645. Typical cognitive-behavioral interventions for patients with generalized anxiety disorder target the worry process with restructuring of anxiety.

646. Repeatedly exposing a patient with OCD to previously avoided cues without performing compulsive acts has little impact on anxiety.

647. CBT is less effective than is medication for OCD.

648. Exposure-based interventions remain the mainstays of CBT interventions for specific phobias.

649. Systematic desensitization relies on the use of a hypnotic induction to reduce anxiety day by day.

For questions 650 to 654, match the stages and the process for readiness for undertaking behavioral change in the left column with the statements in the right column.

650. Pre-contemplation

651. Contemplation

652. Preparation

653. Action

654. Maintenance

a. No interest in behavioral change; denies impact of behavior on health

b. Preparing to change; is ready for a lifestyle intervention with little help

c. Has changed health behaviors quite some time ago and is not at major risk for relapse

d. Thinks about changing health behavior; low confidence in ability to change, has fears and concerns about changing

e. Has just recently changed health behavior but can return to old behaviors fairly easily (relapse)

Questions 655 to 659 are *true-false* questions.

655. Most physicians have received training and have experience in behavior intervention counseling skills.

656. Patients view discussion about prevention as evidence of a caring and concerned physician.

657. Physicians are reimbursed for procedures and management of acute illness of complex severity at higher levels than for cognitive services of a preventive nature.

658. By and large, most medical practices are not organized to facilitate behavioral change programs.

659. Compliance and adherence are terms used to describe a patient's behavior in taking medication, following a diet, or executing lifestyle changes on the medical advice of a clinician.

660. Which of the following statements regarding noncompliance is *false?*

a. 10 to 20% of patients fail to keep appointments they make in the primary care setting.
b. 30 to 40% of patients fail to keep appointments when the appointment is made for them.
c. The longer the interval between a scheduled appointment and the appointment date, the more likely it is that the appointment will not be kept.
d. Patients stop taking their medication after several days 50% of the time.
e. Patients fail to fill their prescriptions 30 to 35% of the time.

661. Which of the following statements regarding noncompliance is *false?*

a. Patients do not complete a 10-day course of treatment 75 to 80% of the time.
b. Patients do not comply with long-term treatments 75 to 80% of the time.
c. Compliance problems increase with the duration of an illness.
d. Patients do not follow modest dietary recommendations 70% of the time.
e. Patients do not stop using tobacco products 90 to 95% of the time after being advised to do so.

662. *True-false.* Ordering serum or urine drug levels as a means of determining a patient's level of compliance with drug taking may compromise the patient's trust in the doctor-patient relationship.

663. Improving visit attendance rates may be facilitated by each of the following *except*

a. Patients should receive reminders by phone or mail before a visit
b. If a visit is missed, the patient should be telephoned
c. Whenever possible, the office wait should be kept to a minimum
d. Keep information about what is wrong with a patient from him or her
e. Follow-up appointments should be made in the office at the conclusion of a visit

Questions 664 to 666 are *true-false* questions.

664. Cigarette smoking is the single most preventable cause of death in the United States.

665. Roughly one-fourth to one-third of American smokers have quit.

666. Approximately two-thirds of those who quit smoking resume smoking within 1 month.

667. Obstacles commonly observed in the process of smoking cessation that impede smoking cessation attempts include each of the following *except*

a. Weight gain
b. Nicotine withdrawal symptoms
c. Availability of acupuncturists
d. Dependence on cigarettes to deal with stress and unpleasant feelings
e. Co-morbid psychiatric symptoms or syndromes

668. Nicotine withdrawal symptoms include each of the following *except*

a. Craving
b. Increased sleep
c. Irritability
d. Impatience
e. Increased appetite

Questions 669 to 670 are *true-false* questions.

669. Nicotine withdrawal symptoms begin within 1 hour of smoking cessation and may persist for several days.

670. Antidepressant treatment in patients with depressive disorders has been shown to improve quit rates.

671. Nicotine toxicity can occur with excessive use of nicotine chewing gum, and includes each of the following *except*

a. Dyspepsia
b. Vivid dreams
c. Hiccups
d. Sleepiness
e. Dizziness

Questions 672 to 678 are *true-false* questions.

672. Body mass index (BMI) is calculated by the formula: weight in pounds divided by height in inches.

673. The amount of activity or exercise is more important than the type or intensity of exercise for weight loss.

674. Exercising at a lower intensity for a longer period of time is not as beneficial as exercising at a higher intensity for a shorter period of time.

675. A difficult patient is almost always an individual with a personality disorder.

676. Patients with personality disorders often become troublesome by virtue of their severe dependency in interpersonal relationships.

677. Individuals with borderline personality disorder often have difficulty tolerating distance and closeness.

678. Difficult patients' problems with interpersonal closeness always involve the physician.

679. The tendency of a personality-disordered patient to see one caregiver as omnipotent and omniscient while devaluating and denigrating another is called
a. Projective identification
b. Splitting
c. Entitlement
d. Manipulativeness
e. Denial

680. The defense mechanism of a personality-disordered patient that is opposite to idealization, seen when the patient dumps pathology, particularly envy and rage, onto the physician is called

a. Projective identification
b. Splitting
c. Entitlement
d. Manipulativeness
e. Denial

Questions 681 to 688 are *true-false* questions.

681. Entitlement can be seen as an emotionally deprived individual's attempt to collect now what he or she should have gotten "back then."

682. In limit-setting confrontations with manipulative, entitled patients, the physician should assault the patient's sense of entitlement to clarify expectations for appropriate behavior.

683. Denial should be confronted routinely in the medical setting so that patients and physicians can collaborate on a treatment plan.

684. Entitled demanders tend to have a deep sense of profound defectiveness and ugliness despite their outward bluster.

685. Anxious clingers generally induce a feeling of aversion in the physician caring for them.

686. When working with the paranoid individual, it helps to remind the patient that you as the physician are worthy of his or her trust.

687. If the physician feels depressed and de-skilled by a patient's continued and seemingly deliberate failure to comply with and to respond to treatment, the patient is probably an entitled demander.

688. From the outset, dependent clingers need to have gentle but firm limits set on their dependent behaviors and attempts at seduction.

689. Which of the following conditions is the *least* likely to require a referral to a psychiatrist?

a. A psychotic disorder
b. A substance-related disorder
c. A sexual and gender-identity disorder
d. An eating disorder
e. An anxiety disorder

Questions 690 to 696 are *true-false* questions.

690. Referral by a primary care provider to a mental health provider should be viewed as an indication that the primary care provider wants to help the patient, not as an accusation or indication of abandonment.

691. Referral by a PCP to a colleague who is a psychiatrist should be discouraged because of the potential appearance of cronyism.

692. It is wise for a PCP to avoid telling a patient the true reason for a referral to a psychiatrist because of concerns about the patient's potential reaction.

693. The PCP should never insist on the patient's referral to a psychiatrist.

694. The prevalence of depression in primary care settings is greater than the prevalence of hypertension.

695. The lifetime prevalence for anxiety disorders in the general population is less than 10%.

696. Two-thirds of patients with undiagnosed depression have more than or equal to six visits per year with a PCP for somatic complaints.

697. Barriers to diagnosis and treatment of psychiatric disorders in primary care settings include each of the following *except*

a. Patients may deny the presence of depressive symptoms and focus instead on somatic complaints.
b. Fear of referral to a psychiatrist may be due to stigma and shame.
c. The belief that the physician has not understood their distress may lead to inaccurate treatment.
d. Patients may fear that psychiatric referral will lead to abandonment by the PCP.
e. Patients may believe that psychiatric illness is untreatable.

698. Which of the following would be *least* likely to be barriers to a PCP's appropriate referral to a psychiatrist?

a. There is often a lack of time to make an accurate diagnosis.
b. Uncertainty may exist as to how to make an appropriate referral.
c. The PCP may believe that one successful referral may lead to a stampede of other patients to psychiatrists.
d. A lack of knowledge may exist about appropriate diagnosis, drugs, and duration of treatment.
e. The PCP may not want to stigmatize a patient.

699. *True-false.* In some collaborative management models of care, patients alternate visits to PCPs and psychiatrists within the same clinic setting.

700. Characteristics of a model primary care psychiatry clinic include each of the following *except*

a. Availability
b. Adequate staffing
c. Rotating blocks of consulting time
d. On-site communication with PCPs
e. Good communication skills among staff

Questions 701 to 707 are *true-false* questions.

701. Psychoanalytic psychotherapy deals with unconscious conflicts, repressed feelings, family issues from early in a patient's life, and difficulties with current relationships.

702. Behavior therapy is usually unstructured and revolves around learning how to relax in multiple environments.

703. Cognitive therapy is based on the assumption that negative thoughts promote depression or anxiety.

704. Interpersonal therapy deals with unconscious conflicts, repressed feelings, and family issues from early in a patient's life.

705. Group therapy rarely involves groups with homogeneous conditions for a time-limited treatment.

706. Informed consent relies on obtaining a patient's signature on a form for the medical record.

707. Informed consent is a process through which the physician gets the permission of a patient or a substituted decision-maker to provide treatment to that patient.

708. Which of the following statements regarding informed consent is *false?*
a. The patient must be competent; that is, have the capacity to make decisions.
b. Informed consent cannot be obtained from a health care proxy.
c. The patient must be given enough information to make an informed decision.
d. The patient must make the decision voluntarily.
e. The patient may need to be assessed several times between provision of the information and when the patient is asked to make a decision.

Questions 709 to 722 are *true-false* questions.

709. Informed consent is a risk management tool.

710. A physician who obtains informed consent in a reasonable way is less likely to be perceived as arrogant and deserving of a lawsuit by distressed patients if an adverse outcome develops.

711. When a competent patient wishes to pass the right to make a decision to a family member or to the physician, the patient may do so.

712. Informed consent is a legal, not an ethical obligation of physicians.

713. Autonomy is the patient's right to make his or her own decisions regardless of what the physician or society believes is the best choice.

714. The patient's wishes regarding decisions about his or her care must be followed even if it means the patient will die.

715. Beneficence is the physician's obligation to do what is in the best interest of the patient.

716. Only a psychiatrist can declare a patient to be incompetent.

717. Less capacity is required for low-risk treatments with a high likelihood of a good result than for treatments with a higher level of risk or when the results are less likely to be favorable.

718. Clinical assessments of capacity impact a patient's legal status.

719. A legal declaration of incompetence strips a person of certain rights and privileges normally accorded to adults, such as making treatment decisions, making contracts, or executing a will.

720. The conclusion that a patient lacks the capacity to give informed consent requires the choice of an alternative decision-maker except in an emergency or when the patient has a valid advance directive.

721. Testamentary capacity is the capacity to execute a will.

722. Testimonial capacity is the capacity to serve as a witness in court.

723. When a physician evaluates a patient's capacity to make treatment decisions, each of the following questions is crucial *except*

a. Does the patient express a preference?
b. Is the patient able to attain a factual understanding of the information provided?
c. Is the patient able to appreciate the seriousness of the condition and the consequences of accepting or refusing treatment?
d. Can the patient manipulate the information provided in a rational fashion as to how a decision that follows is logical from the information in the control of the individual's personal beliefs, experience, and condition?
e. Does the patient have minor children?

Questions 724 to 726 are *true-false* questions.

724. Patients who are unable to express a preference are presumed to lack decision-making capacity.

725. Disagreement with the treating clinician and his or her recommendations in and of itself is not a basis for judging that a patient is irrational.

726. The professional standard is the amount of information that the average patient would need to make a decision in the same circumstance.

727. Which of the following pieces of information is *not* essential to provide to a patient in most jurisdictions?

a. The nature of the condition to be treated and the treatment proposed
b. The cost of the treatment to be recommended
c. The nature and probability of the risks associated with the treatment
d. The alternative treatments available, including no treatment
e. The inability to predict the result of the treatment as well as the likelihood of irreversibility of the procedure, if applicable

Questions 728 to 742 are *true-false* questions.

728. Informed consent is not required for all medical treatments.

729. In an emergency, informed consent need not be obtained.

730. If a patient's physical or mental condition will deteriorate as a direct result of the process of providing information, informed consent may be deferred under the doctrine of therapeutic privilege.

731. The patient or decision-maker may withdraw consent at any point during the course of treatment.

732. It is not necessary to document the questions asked by the patient to indicate that the patient was involved in the decision-making process.

733. In most states, involuntary commitment of a patient allows for the treatment of a patient against his or her will.

734. Civil commitment is considered to be an act of the state because it occurs under the authority of the state.

735. Lawsuits for deprivation of civil rights, false imprisonment, and negligence can arise from improper civil commitment.

736. The need for treatment of a psychiatric condition, even in the absence of dangerousness, is sufficient to permit involuntary commitment.

737. All adults, even those with mental illness, are presumed to be competent.

738. The presumption of competency persists until a psychiatrist declares a person to be incompetent.

739. The assessment of risk should begin, but not end, with questioning the patient about thoughts of self-injury.

740. In many states, the law imposes a duty on clinicians to take steps to protect the safety of third parties against whom a patient issues threats.

741. When a patient refuses psychiatric care, it is helpful to ask if the patient's explanation for the refusal suggests a rational decision or incompetence.

742. The *Diagnostic and Statistical Manual of Psychiatry,* Fourth Edition, for Primary Care (*DSM-IV PC*) is a manual organized around symptoms but not diagnoses.

743. Each of the following are reasons that PCPs should screen for psychiatric disorders *except*

a. The estimated prevalence of psychiatric disorders in primary care approaches 30%.
b. Most patients with a mental illness present to primary care settings.
c. Psychiatric disorders are under-recognized and under-treated in the medical setting.
d. Unrecognized psychiatric illness can be disabling.
e. Screening without adequate education may stigmatize the patient.

744. Each of the following are reasons that PCPs should screen for psychiatric disorders *except*

a. Direct and indirect costs of untreated mental disorders are substantial.
b. Lack of recognition and treatment is associated with increased use of medical services.
c. There is a risk of treating false positives if screening is used improperly.
d. Recognition and treatment improve morbidity of other medical conditions.
e. Existing screens for psychiatric illness are as effective as many common medical tests.

745. Elements of an appropriate screen include each of the following *except*

a. It is fast.
b. It is inexpensive.
c. It is valid and reliable.
d. It is comprehensive.
e. It is in a language that the patient understands.

For questions 746 to 750, match the name of the screening instrument in the left column with the characteristics of the screen in the right column.

746. General Health Questionnaire (GHQ)

747. Primary Care Evaluation of
Mental Disorders (Prime
MD)

748. Symptom Driven Diagnostic
System for Primary Care
(SDDS-PC)

749. Screener

750. Beck Depression Inventory
(BDI)

a. A two-part screening instrument of
26 yes-no questions for five types
of psychiatric illness: mood, anxiety, somatoform disorders, alcohol,
and eating disorders

b. A 44- or 96-item questionnaire
screen for 15 diagnoses in five
areas: mood, anxiety, somatoform
disorders, substance abuse, and
eating disorders

c. An internationally tested symptom
checklist describing both positive
and negative feelings with 28- or
30-item versions useful in the
medical setting with four sub-
scales: anxiety, severe depression,
social dysfunction, and psychotic
symptoms

d. A two-part, 26-item scale for six
psychiatric disorders and suicidal
ideation, major depression, panic,
GAD, OCD, alcohol, and drug dependence piloted with a 1-800
telephone number for computer
analysis

e. A 13- or 21-item self-report scale
investigating neurovegetative, cognitive, and mood symptoms

For questions 751 to 755, match the name of the screening instrument in the left column with the characteristics of screen in the right column.

751. Center for Epidemiologic Studies Depression Scale (CESD)

752. Zung Self-Rating Depression Scale (SDS)

753. CAGE

754. Mini Mental State Examination (MMSE)

755. Short Information Memory Concentration Test (IMCT)

a. A six-item test aimed at discriminating between patients with organic brain syndromes and normal elderly patients

b. A 20-item screen useful in primary care settings to measure present levels of depression and duration of depression

c. A four-item screen for exploration of the extent and pattern of drinking

d. A 20-item self-report scale with graded responses of 1 through 4 favored by NIMH on its National Depression Screening Day

e. A 30-point test of orientation, registration, attention, calculation, recall, and language that screens for dementia and organic brain syndromes

756. The limbic system is thought to regulate each of the following functions *except*

a. Gender roles
b. Territoriality
c. Executive functions
d. Bonding
e. The **four F's: fear, feeding, flight, and fornication**

Questions 757 to 771 are *true-false* questions.

757. Typically, when a patient presents with psychological unresponsiveness, the patient will have his or her eyes closed and the examiner will not be able to open them due to conscious resistance by the patient.

758. In the psychologically unresponsive patient, if the patient's arm is lifted above his or her face and then dropped, it will always miss the face.

759. Boundary crossings are more serious than boundary violations.

760. What constitutes a boundary crossing or violation is determined in part by both the nature of the action and the setting in which it occurs.

761. The nature of certain personality traits (e.g., dependency) and disorders (e.g., borderline personality disorder) may lead patients to actively challenge the boundaries of the relationship in a search for interpersonal fulfillment that they may not have obtained outside the treatment setting.

762. The American Medical Association's Council on Ethical and Judicial Affairs has passed a rule that prohibits physician-patient sexual contact regardless of the physician's specialty.

763. The American Psychiatric Association has adopted a guideline that declares it unethical to have a sexual relationship with a current patient, but not with a former patient.

764. In some states, it is a criminal offense for a physician to have a sexual relationship with a patient.

765. Business dealings between a physician and a patient can impinge on the objectivity of a physician in dealing with a patient, and are not recommended.

766. The use of overly familiar touching or language during a physical examination is not considered to be a boundary crossing.

767. Inappropriate behavior during a physical examination can lead to civil and potentially criminal litigation.

768. Although patients often give gifts to their physicians as a sign of appreciation, accepting valuable gifts can compromise a physician's judgment.

769. At times, boundary violations are a result of the patient's failure to maintain appropriate boundaries in the relationship with a physician.

770. When a physician begins to do things that he or she would not do for other patients, it is an indication that boundaries are being strained.

771. It is neither necessary nor advisable for the physician to discuss boundary violations with the patient if a boundary crossing occurs.

772. When PCPs treat somatizing patients, each of the following strategies has been found useful *except*
a. Scheduling more frequent PCP-patient meetings
b. Insisting that the patient enter group therapy
c. Paying close attention to physical symptoms during visits with the PCP
d. Placing limits on outside referrals
e. Avoiding defining the patient's problem as psychiatric

773. *True-false.* Managed care carve-outs often create a misalignment of incentives between primary care providers and the mental health carve-out company.

774. Medical training encourages behaviors that contribute to burnout. These include each of the following *except*
a. The availability of computerized literature searches
b. Sleep deprivation
c. Repression of feelings
d. Isolation from ordinary social situations
e. Frequent demands by patients and families

775. Which of the following statements regarding the health and mental health of physicians is *false?*
a. In the United States, the number of physicians who suicide annually would fill an average-size medical school class.
b. Female physicians die an average of 10 years earlier than women outside of medicine.
c. Roughly 20% of house officers require a leave of absence during their training secondary to stress-related problems.
d. Substance abuse often leads to physician impairment.
e. PCPs are particularly vulnerable to chemical dependency and psychiatric disorders related to stress.

776. Which of the following is *least* likely to be a source of physician stress and burnout?

a.   Dealing with difficult clinical situations
b.   Developing new roots and social relationships
c.   Having responsibility without authority
d.   Having disrupted marital and social relationships
e.   Having substantial amounts of personal financial debt

777. Manifestations of unmanageable stress in physicians are likely to include each of the following *except*

a.   Exhaustion
b.   Apathy
c.   Lack of dream recall
d.   Anhedonia
e.   Headaches

778. Strategies that have been helpful when dealing with physician stress include each of the following *except*

a.   Talking with a colleague in an attempt to process the experience
b.   Talking over personal history and responses to past stresses
c.   Rehearsing potential problems to predict one's responses to them
d.   Minimizing and denying the dysfunction
e.   Using humor and mutual support

779. Professional consultation for a physician who is overwhelmed and stressed should be considered when each of the following is present *except*

a.   Depression is evident
b.   Suicidal ideation has developed
c.   A tic has developed
d.   Rage is inappropriately expressed
e.   Reckless behavior has developed

780. The inability to maintain a coherent stream of thought or action is defined as which of the following?

a.   Delirium
b.   Drowsiness
c.   Stupor
d.   Confusion
e.   Coma

781. Incomplete arousal to painful stimuli is defined as which of the following?

a. Delirium
b. Drowsiness
c. Stupor
d. Confusion
e. Coma

For questions 782 to 786, match the type of respiratory effort in the left column with its characteristics listed in the right column.

782. Cheyne-Stokes respiration
783. Central neurogenic hyperventilation
784. Apneustic breathing
785. Ataxic breathing
786. Depressed breathing

a. Breathing with a prolonged inspiratory phase followed by apnea
b. Periods of hyperventilation that gradually diminish to apnea of variable duration; breathing then resumes and gradually increases to hyperventilation
c. Shallow, slow, ineffective breathing
d. Continuous, rapid, regular, deep respirations at a rate of about 25 per minute
e. Chaotic respirations

787. Coma with hyperventilation is seen in each of the following conditions *except*

a. Diabetic ketoacidosis
b. Respiratory acidosis
c. Uremia
d. Ingestion of organic acids
e. Lactic acidosis

Questions 788 to 789 are *true-false* questions.

788. In hemispheric lesions, the head and eyes deviate toward the lesion and away from the hemiparesis.

789. Reactive pupils indicate an intact midbrain.

790. A unilaterally dilated and unreactive pupil may be caused by each of the following *except*

a. Third nerve compression due to temporal lobe herniation
b. Essential anisocoria
c. Prior injury to the iris
d. Administration of pilocarpine into the eye
e. Administration of a mydriatic agent into the eye

Questions 791 to 794 are *true-false* questions.

791. In the conscious patient, a normal response to irrigation of the tympanic membrane with cold water is nystagmus with tonic deviation of the eyes toward the water infusion, followed by a quick correction movement toward the opposite side.

792. The fast phase of nystagmus in response to irrigation of the tympanic membrane with cold water is mediated by brainstem pathways extending from the vestibular nuclei in the medulla toward the oculomotor nucleus in the midbrain.

793. When the doll's head maneuver is performed in unconscious patients, the reflex is normal or preserved if the eyes move in the orbits in the direction opposite to the rotating head to maintain their position relative to the environment.

794. In psychogenic unresponsiveness, there will be both slow and fast components to the nystagmus associated with ice water calorics.

795. Each of the following statements is associated with classic migraines *except*

a. A visual aura precedes a throbbing headache by 15 to 20 minutes.
b. A throbbing headache intensifies over 1 to 6 hours and typically lasts 6 to 24 hours.
c. A majority of migraine sufferers recall childhood vomiting or motion sickness.
d. Vomiting, nausea, and irritability are common with classic migraines.
e. Onset of the first migraine headache usually occurs between 10 and 30 years of age.

796. Each of the following statements is associated with cluster headaches *except*

a. Cluster headaches are typically unilateral.
b. Cluster headaches are typically described as boring or sharp.
c. Cluster headaches typically last 15 to 120 minutes.
d. Cluster headaches are associated with ipsilateral tearing, facial flushing, nasal stuffiness and Horner's syndrome.
e. Cluster headaches tend to be preceded by a visual aura.

797. Each of the following statements about cluster headaches is true *except*

a. Headaches often occur in clusters occurring daily for three weeks to three months, then remit for months to years.
b. Nausea and vomiting are typically absent with cluster headaches.
c. Headaches are most common late at night or early in the morning.
d. Headaches are often exacerbated by use of alcohol.
e. Women are affected by cluster headaches five times as often as men.

For questions 798 to 802, match the physical finding in the left column with possible etiology for the headache in the right column.

798. Cranial bruit	a. Trigeminal neuralgia
799. Hemiparesis	b. Malignant hypertension
800. Retinal hemorrhage	c. Subarachnoid hemorrhage
801. Trigger point for pain	d. Arteriovenous malformation (AVM)
802. Stiff neck	e. Mass lesion

803. *True-false.* Sumatriptan is effective in ending migraine headaches whether it is given at the onset of migraines or later in the attack.

804. Classes of drugs useful in the prevention of migraines include each of the following *except*

a. TCAs
b. SSRIs
c. NSAIDs
d. Benzodiazepines
e. Beta-blockers

805. Ergotamines are contraindicated in each of the following *except*

a. Renal failure
b. Coronary artery disease
c. Hepatic failure
d. Glaucoma
e. Pregnancy

Questions 806 to 808 are *true-false* questions.

806. The Stanford Binet Test, fourth edition, is a test heavily weighted toward verbal performance that is appropriate for people aged two years to adulthood; it yields mental age and IQ values.

807. Mild mental retardation is associated with an IQ between 70 and 90.

808. Despite Pick's disease degeneration in frontal and temporal poles, it is rare for it to manifest signs of pyramidal tract dysfunction.

809. Each of the following statements about tacrine is true *except*

a. Tacrine is an anticholinesterase agent that may have a modest beneficial effect on the course of Alzheimer's disease.
b. If, during dose escalation, the ALT (also known as the SGPT) doubles, tacrine should be discontinued.
c. Patients who develop clinical jaundice with a total bilirubin level greater than 3 mg/dL should have tacrine discontinued and not be re-challenged with it.
d. Tacrine is generally started at doses of 10 mg PO q.i.d. for 6 weeks.
e. If the ALT remains less than or equal to three times the upper limit of normal, the dose should be increased to 160 mg QD.

Questions 810 to 811 are *true-false* questions.

810. The MELAS syndrome is characterized by a mitochondrial encephalopathy, lactic acidosis, and stroke-like episodes.

811. Dysequilibrium is defined as a sense of imbalance, unsteadiness, or drunkenness with vertigo occurring in patients who have a mismatch of inputs from the systems subserving spatial orientation.

812. Standard tests of dizziness include each of the following *except*

a. Checking for orthostatic hypotension
b. Vigorous hyperventilation for three minutes
c. Sudden turns when walking, or spinning the patient while standing
d. An EEG
e. Valsalva maneuvers that can exacerbate vertigo associated with cranio-vertebral junction anomalies

813. Central causes of dizziness include each of the following *except*

a. Brainstem ischemia
b. Multiple sclerosis
c. Posterior fossa tumors
d. Ménière's disease
e. Basilar migraine

814. Peripheral causes of dizziness include each of the following *except*

a. Motion sickness
b. Vestibular neuronitis
c. Benign positional vertigo
d. Hyperventilation
e. Labyrinthitis

815. Drugs used in the symptomatic treatment of vertigo include each of the following *except*

a. Meclizine
b. Diphenhydramine
c. Hydroxyzine
d. Verapamil
e. Scopolamine

816. Classes of drugs used to treat vertigo include each of the following *except*

a. Antihistamines
b. Anticholinergics
c. Phenothiazines
d. Sympathomimetics
e. Calcium channel blockers

Questions 817 to 818 are *true-false* questions.

817. In patients with chronic back pain in whom the neurological exam is normal, depression is a common finding.

818. Epilepsy is a state of recurrent seizures.

819. Generalized seizures include each of the following *except*

a. Petit mal seizures
b. Grand mal seizures
c. Myoclonic epilepsy
d. Complex partial seizures
e. Febrile seizures

820. *True-false.* There is no diagnostic test that can reliably diagnose or exclude epilepsy.

821. Each of the following statements about absence or petit mal seizures is true *except*

a. They are associated with three per second generalized spike and slow waves seen on the EEG.
b. They typically begin between the ages of 4 and 8.
c. The patient is usually aware of attacks of petit mal seizures.
d. Attacks are usually 5 to 10 seconds in duration.
e. They are often successfully managed with ethosuximide.

822. Drugs known to elevate the blood level of phenytoin or to increase the risk of toxic side-effects include each of the following *except*

a. Coumadin
b. Diazepam
c. Estrogen
d. Carbamazepine
e. Methylphenidate

823. Criteria for brain death include each of the following *except*

a. Absence of endogenous or exogenous toxins
b. Unresponsiveness to noxious stimuli
c. An isoelectric EEG
d. A body temperature greater than 103° Fahrenheit
e. Absent cranial reflexes

824. *True-false.* The Jarisch-Herxheimer reaction is a febrile response believed to be caused by acute primary infection with the treponema that causes syphilis.

825. The Jarisch-Herxheimer reaction is characterized by each of the following *except*

a. Chills
b. Myalgias
c. Headache
d. Hypertension
e. Tachypnea

Questions 826 to 827 are *true-false* questions.

826. Pseudoseizures are most common in patients with true epilepsy.

827. With arteriovenous malformations (AVMs), a chronic headache is often present prior to hemorrhage.

828. The most common brain tumor listed below in adults is

a. Malignant glioma
b. Meningioma
c. Schwannoma
d. Pituitary adenoma
e. Craniopharyngioma

829. Complications of whole brain radiation therapy for malignant gliomas in patients who have survived two years or more include each of the following *except*

a. White matter changes
b. Progressive cognitive impairment
c. Cerebral atrophy
d. Hair loss
e. Hypertension

830. Each of the following statements regarding chronic subdural hematomas (SDHs) is true *except*

a. Chronic SDHs may follow trivial trauma.
b. A gradual drift into stupor or coma may occur following chronic SDHs.
c. SDHs involve a collection of blood between the dura and the underlying brain.
d. Mental status changes secondary to SDHs may simulate dementia.
e. As the interval lengthens from the time of injury, the CT density of the hematoma changes from hypodense to isodense to hyperdense.

831. The medical treatment of patients with increased intracranial pressure secondary to head injury is *least* likely to be of benefit with which of the following?

a. Elevation of the head of the bed
b. Ventricular drainage
c. Mannitol
d. Hyperventilation
e. Steroids

832. Each of the following statements about multiple sclerosis (MS) is true *except*

a. No specific laboratory test can confirm the diagnosis of multiple sclerosis.
b. Physical examination is consistent with multiple lesions in central nervous system white matter.
c. Oligoclonal bands of IGG can be demonstrated in 25 to 35% of patients with multiple sclerosis.
d. The CSF is abnormal in the majority of patients, often with pleocytosis.
e. Nearly 75% of patients with multiple sclerosis have elevated CSF gamma globulin levels.

833. Each of the following is true about multiple sclerosis patients *except*

a. An increase in CSF myelin protein may confirm an acute attack.
b. Visual evoked responses are abnormal in approximately 80% of patients with definite MS and 50% with probable MS.
c. MRI and CT scans are roughly equivalent in the detection of CNS demyelination.
d. Brainstem auditory evoked responses are abnormal in approximately 50% of patients with definite MS and 20% with probable MS.
e. Somatosensory evoked responses are abnormal in 70% of those with either probable or definite MS.

834. Each of the following is associated with multiple sclerosis (MS) *except*

a. Fatigue
b. Heat sensitivity
c. Vitamin B_{12} deficiency
d. Optic neuritis
e. Spasticity

835. Overly rapid correction of hyponatremia is associated with which of the following?

a. Subarachnoid hemorrhage
b. Hyperglycemia
c. Abdominal pain
d. Central pontine myelinolysis
e. Hypotension

836. Lead poisoning is manifested by each of the following *except*

a. Personality change
b. Lethargy
c. Diarrhea
d. Irritability
e. Ataxia

837. Each of the following statements regarding carbon monoxide poisoning is true *except*

a. It is the most frequent cause of death by poisoning in the United States.
b. It presents with hypoxia without cyanosis.
c. Subacute demyelinization of white matter develops one to two months after carbon monoxide poisoning.
d. Choreoathetosis, myoclonus, and Parkinson-like symptoms may follow carbon monoxide poisoning.
e. Hyperbaric oxygen administration is beneficial for those with severe carbon monoxide poisoning.

838. Each of the following statements regarding physostigmine is true *except*

a. Physostigmine injection may serve as a diagnostic test to confirm anticholinergic ingestion.
b. If no anticholinergics are present, physostigmine may result in bradycardia, salivation, lacrimation, and pupillary constriction.
c. Its effects can be counteracted with atropine.
d. If given in excessive amounts, its anticholinergic effects can be toxic.
e. Given intravenously, its duration of action is one to two hours.

839. Each of the following statements regarding vitamin B_{12} deficiency is true *except*

a. It may result from an acquired defect in intestinal absorption of the vitamin due to intrinsic factor deficiency.
b. Occupational exposure to nitrous oxide can duplicate the clinical features of cobalamin deficiency.
c. Vitamin B_{12} deficiency may be manifested by subacute combined degeneration of the spinal cord.
d. It may be marked by personality change and dementia.
e. Folate and cobalamin should be administered immediately following the diagnosis of vitamin B_{12} deficiency.

840. Each of the following agents can treat spasticity *except*

a. Diazepam
b. Baclofen
c. Dantrolene
d. Botulinum toxin
e. Amitriptyline

841. *True-false.* Bromocriptine is a dopamine receptor antagonist predominantly affecting D_2 receptors.

842. Each of the following statements regarding Huntington's disease is true *except*

a. It is an inherited autosomal dominant disease.
b. Chorea and athetosis may be present.
c. Depression can be seen.
d. The genetic defect is a repeated replication sequence on chromosome 11.
e. Treatment with dopamine depleters or receptor blockade is helpful in the early stages.

843. Each of the following statements regarding Wilson's disease is true *except*

a. It is a rare autosomal dominant disorder.
b. It is characterized by progressive liver and neurologic disease.
c. It is characterized by Kayser-Fleischer rings of the cornea.
d. Younger patients have rapid progression of either athetosis or rigidity and dystonia.
e. Treatment with D-penicillamine retards the progression of the disease.

844. Neuropsychological testing is often used as an adjunct in the assessment of each of the following *except*

a. Dementia
b. Depression
c. Neurological disease
d. Neurosurgical interventions
e. Debilitation

845. Neuropsychological testing can be complicated or impractical in each of the following *except*

a. The intubated patient
b. The visually impaired patient
c. The aphasic patient
d. The aprosodic patient
e. The quadriplegic patient

846. The Wisconsin Card Sorting Test is used for the assessment of

a. Parietal lobe function
b. Temporal lobe function
c. Frontal lobe function
d. Occipital lobe function
e. Cerebellar function

847. The Mini Mental State Examination assesses each of the following *except*

a. Ability to register new information
b. Orientation
c. Recall
d. Language
e. Executive function

848. The Wechsler Adult Intelligence Scale (WAIS) is a standardized and widely used test that assesses each of the following *except*

a. Comprehension
b. Abstraction
c. Coordination
d. Interpretation of proverbs
e. Planning

849. The Minnesota Multiphasic Personality Inventory (MMPI) is a widely used inventory with each of the following features *except*

a. Three validity scales
b. 10 clinical scales
c. A conversion V pattern in multiple sclerosis patients
d. 566 items
e. A multiple choice format

850. Right parietal lesions may lead to impairment in each of the following *except*

a. Double simultaneous stimulation
b. Clock drawing
c. Emotional expressivity
d. Line bisection
e. Executive function

851. Neuropsychological testing can be used for each of the following *except*

a. To obtain a baseline level of performance
b. To measure decline or improvement from prior testing
c. To rule out an underlying seizure disorder
d. To assess beginning dementia or depression
e. To help plan rehabilitation

852. The term *hypnosis* was first coined by which of the following?

a. James Braid
b. Jean-Martin Charcot
c. Benjamin Franklin
d. Franz Anton Mesmer
e. Sigmund Freud

853. Which of the following statements is *not* true for hypnosis?

a. It is a state of sleep.
b. It involves a state of heightened concentration.
c. It is used to facilitate psychotherapy.
d. It is used to control pain.
e. It is used to modify behavior patterns.

854. Hypnosis is *least* likely to be successful in which of the following patients?

a. Histrionic patients
b. Demented patients
c. Paranoid patients
d. Patients who dissociate
e. Pain patients

855. Hypnosis is often used for each of the following reasons *except*

a. To enhance the patient's control
b. To facilitate denial
c. To uncover material the patient has repressed
d. To alter the patient's symptoms
e. To alter the patient's attitude

856. Hypnosis is relatively *contraindicated* in which type of patient?

a. The depressed patient
b. The paranoid patient
c. The demented patient
d. The pain patient
e. The patient who dissociates

857. The prevalence of major depression in cancer centers is approximately

a. One percent
b. Three percent
c. Six percent
d. 12%
e. 24%

858. Thoughts of suicide are found in what percentage of patients at the time of receiving a diagnosis of cancer?

a. One percent
b. Five percent
c. 10%
d. 20%
e. 30%

859. Anti-emetic treatment options for chemotherapy-induced nausea include each of the following *except*

a. Haloperidol
b. Metoclopramide
c. Ondansetron
d. Dexamethasone
e. Morphine

860. The diagnosis *least* likely to be associated with depressed mood in a cancer patient is

a. Brain metastases
b. Hypothyroidism
c. Treatment with interferon
d. Liver dysfunction
e. Hypocalcemia

861. The prevalence of adjustment disorders in cancer centers is approximately

a. Five percent
b. 15%
c. 25%
d. 35%
e. 45%

862. Treatment for anxiety in the cancer patient includes each of the following *except*

a. Benzodiazepines
b. Neuroleptics
c. Hypnosis
d. Stimulants
e. Behavioral management

863. Paraneoplastic syndromes are most common with which of the following?

a. Pancreatic cancer
b. Gliomas
c. Small cell lung cancer
d. Lymphomas
e. Leukemia

864. A 33-year-old man dependent on heroin is admitted to orthopedic surgery with septic arthritis. He is considered by most of the staff to be a manipulative sociopath who frequently threatens to leave the hospital before completing antibiotic treatment. In the opinion of the psychiatric consultant asked to assess the patient's decision-making capacity, the staff appears to be unusually invested in the patient's staying in the hospital to complete treatment. This is likely to be an example of which of the following defense mechanisms?

a. Projection
b. Projective identification
c. Identification
d. Reaction formation
e. Displacement

865. In a heroin-dependent patient, which of the following signs and symptoms of opiate withdrawal is the *most* reliable?

a. Myalgias and arthralgias
b. Dilated pupils
c. Lacrimation
d. Abdominal pain
e. Rhinorrhea

866. Each of the following statements about the competency evaluation is correct *except*

a. A patient's capacity to make medical decisions can change over the course of hospitalization.
b. Standards for competency to accept treatment and to refuse treatment are the same.
c. Competency is a legal term and thus is appropriately determined only by a judge, not by a physician.
d. Incompetency is not a valid indication for involuntary commitment to a psychiatric hospital.
e. A patient must be able to state in some fashion a clear decision regarding his or her care that is stable over time in order to be considered competent.

867. Each of the following symptoms and signs are typical of opiate withdrawal *except*

a. Miotic pupils
b. Lacrimation
c. Rhinorrhea
d. Abdominal pain
e. Myalgias

868. Each of the following conditions are manifestations of tertiary syphilis *except*

a. Tabes dorsalis
b. Aortitis
c. General paresis
d. Mucocutaneous rash
e. Meningovascular disease

869. The Argyll-Robertson pupil is a manifestation of neurosyphilis. It is characterized by

a. Reaction to light, but failure to accommodate
b. Accommodation, but failure to react to light
c. Failure both to accommodate and to react to light
d. Absence of consensual reaction to light
e. None of the above

Questions 870 to 873 are *true-false* questions.

870. The VDRL test is a nonspecific serum test for syphilis.

871. The RPR test can be positive in certain auto-immune disorders in the absence of treponemal infection.

872. The FTA-ABS test is a specific test for syphilis.

873. The CSF VDRL test can be falsely negative in cases of neurosyphilis.

874. Each of the following symptoms and signs is consistent with the diagnosis of general paresis *except*

a. Personality change
b. Argyll-Robertson pupil
c. Hyporeflexia
d. Affective change
e. Speech change

For questions 875 to 881, match the personality type in the left column with the presumptive intrapsychic meaning of the illness to the patient in the right column.

875. Oral

876. Compulsive

877. Hysterical

878. Masochistic

879. Narcissistic

880. Schizoid

881. Paranoid

a. Threat of intrusion
b. Deserved punishment for worthlessness
c. Threat of loss of self-control
d. Threat of abandonment
e. Threat of attack
f. Threat to self-image of autonomy and perfection
g. Threat to masculinity or femininity

882. Criteria for borderline personality disorder include each of the following *except*

a. Chronic feelings of emptiness or boredom
b. Recurrent suicidal threats or gestures
c. Frequent displays of temper
d. A lack of ability to function as a responsible parent
e. A pattern of unstable interpersonal relationships

883. Which of the following is *not* true about antisocial personality disorder?

a. It is manifested by a pattern of irresponsible behavior.
b. It is associated with evidence of a conduct disorder.
c. It has a male-female ratio of 3 to 1.
d. It has a familial linkage.
e. It is often helped by insight-oriented psychotherapy.

884. The concept of there being seven distinct personality types associated with medical illness is attributed to

a. Franz Alexander
b. Helen Dunbar
c. Thomas Hackett and Avery Weisman
d. Ralph Kahana and Greta Bibring
e. Milton Viederman

885. Which of the following is *not* an essential part of the case formulation in the psychiatric consultation note on a medical-surgical patient?

a. A psychiatric diagnosis
b. A discussion of possible etiology
c. A concise summary of psychiatric symptoms
d. Use of psychiatric terminology
e. Provision of a psychodynamic formulation

886. Which of the following is *not* typically a function of the psychiatric consultant?

a. Evaluation of the mental status of the patient
b. Arranging a transfer of the patient to a psychiatric service
c. Evaluation of capacity and competency
d. Making a diagnosis based solely on data in the medical record
e. Giving advice on the use of psychotropic agents

887. Assessment of language does not include determination of

a. Rate of speech
b. Dysarthria
c. Aphasia
d. Speech latency
e. Interpretation of proverbs

888. The psychiatric consultation note on a general hospital inpatient is *not*

a. A legal record
b. An official doctor-to-doctor communication
c. A supplement to a doctor's memory
d. A document that belongs to the hospital
e. Routinely submitted to third-party payers for reimbursement

889. The mental status examination does *not* include

a. A general description of the patient's appearance
b. An assessment of language
c. The results of the Mini Mental State Exam
d. An assessment of insight and judgment
e. An assessment of competency

890. The psychiatric consultant should *not*

a. Determine the question being asked
b. Establish the urgency of the consult
c. Call doctors at other hospitals to clarify information
d. Review old records
e. Provide an extensive list of general recommendations

891. The psychiatric consultant should *not*

a. Recommend psychopharmacological treatment
b. Recommend psychotherapeutic treatment
c. Provide legal advice
d. Recommend laboratory tests
e. Provide formulations of psychopathology

892. Psychiatric consultants do *not* commonly

a. Evaluate competency
b. Evaluate and treat agitated patients
c. Evaluate and treat agitated family members
d. Assess suicide risk
e. Evaluate and treat delirium

893. In general, the psychiatric consultant should *not*

a. Provide a range of options to the treatment team
b. Review previous consultation notes
c. Document in detail the report of the consultation in the medical record
d. Discharge the patient
e. Follow the patient until the problem is resolved

894. Common reasons for emergent psychiatric consultations include each of the following *except*

a. Evaluation of competency
b. Assessment of a patient wishing to leave against medical advice
c. Evaluation of suicidality
d. Evaluation of agitation
e. Evaluation of dementia

895. Primary functions of liaison psychiatrists include each of the following *except*

a. Rounding with the medical team
b. Resolving staff conflicts
c. Doing consultations with patients
d. Teaching psychiatric skills to the medical team
e. Performing clinical research

896. The former director of the Psychiatric Education Branch at the NIMH who supported the growth of consultation-liaison programs in the 1960s was

a. Bish Lipowski
b. James Strain
c. James Eaton
d. Avery Weisman
e. Patrick McKegney

897. The mental status examination should include each of the following *except*

a. A general description of the patient's appearance
b. Assessment of language
c. Assessment of insight and judgment
d. Assessment of competency
e. Assessment of mood

898. Assessment of language includes examination for

a. Presence of aphasia
b. Presence of aprosodia
c. Presence of dysarthria
d. Ability to repeat phrases
e. Ability to correctly interpret proverbs

899. Recommendations by the psychiatric consultant should address each of the following *except*

a. Psychopharmacological treatment
b. Psychotherapeutic treatment
c. Recommendations for legal management
d. Laboratory tests
e. Formulations of psychopathology

900. Typical reasons for a psychiatric consultation in a general hospital include each of the following *except*

a. Evaluation of competency
b. Evaluation and treatment of an agitated patient
c. Evaluation and treatment of an agitated family member
d. Assessment of suicide risk
e. Evaluation of delirium

901. Which class of drugs is *least* likely to be used in the treatment of delirium?

a. Neuroleptics
b. Benzodiazepines
c. Narcotics
d. Anticholinergic agents
e. Paralytic agents

902. Which of the following abnormalities is *not* typically seen in delirium?

a. Agitation
b. Memory deficits
c. Inattention
d. Aphasia
e. Dysgraphia

903. Agitation is characterized primarily by which of the following?

a. Excessive motor activity
b. Hallucinations
c. Disorientation
d. Mydriasis
e. Memory deficits

904. The incidence of delirium among medical patients in the general hospital is approximately

a. One percent
b. Five percent
c. 10%
d. 25%
e. 50%

905. The incidence of delirium is *highest* among which of the following?

a. Burn patients
b. Cardiac patients
c. Dialysis patients
d. Psychiatric patients
e. Pediatric patients

906. Which of the following drugs is *least* likely to cause delirium?

a. Lidocaine
b. Diphenhydramine
c. Meperidine
d. Cimetidine
e. Erythromycin

907. Which of the following is *not* a primary feature of delirium?

a. Memory deficits
b. Delusions
c. Perceptual disturbances
d. Disorientation
e. Poor attention

908. Which type of EEG recording is *most* often seen in delirium?

a. Diffuse slowing
b. Triphasic delta waves
c. Low-voltage beta waves
d. Spikes
e. A normal EEG recording

909. Which of the following conditions is the *most adverse* effect associated with use of high doses of neuroleptics?

a. Atrial fibrillation
b. Torsade des pointes
c. Tachycardia
d. Hypertension
e. Hyperventilation

910. Life-threatening causes of delirium include each of the following *except*

a. Wernicke's encephalopathy
b. Intracranial hemorrhage
c. Hyperkalemia
d. Hypercalcemia
e. Hypoxia

911. *True-false.* The EEG pattern of triphasic delta waves is most commonly seen among patients in delirium tremens.

912. Delirium is *most* often associated with which of the following?

a. Irreversible organic mental changes
b. Impaired long-term memory
c. Fluctuations in cognition and behavior
d. Neologisms
e. Systematic delusions

913. Possible causes of secondary mania include each of the following *except*

a. Use of corticosteroids
b. CNS neoplasms
c. Temporal lobe seizures
d. Schizophrenia
e. Use of AZT

914. Which of the drugs listed is *least* often associated with the onset of delirium?

a. Lidocaine
b. Diphenhydramine
c. Meperidine
d. Cimetidine
e. Sertraline

915. Normeperidine toxicity *most* often leads to which of the following?

a. Somnolence
b. Aphasia
c. Renal failure
d. Congestive heart failure
e. Myoclonus

916. The risk of acute extrapyramidal side-effects from use of neuroleptics is *highest* with

a. Intramuscular administration
b. Intravenous administration
c. Oral administration
d. Low-potency agents
e. Long-lasting agents

917. Signs and symptoms of anticholinergic delirium include each of the following *except*

a. Dry skin
b. Tachycardia
c. Urinary retention
d. Diminished bowel sounds
e. Miosis

918. In the year 2000, approximately what percentage of the U.S. population was at least 65 years of age?

a. 10%
b. 20%
c. 30%
d. 40%
e. 50%

919. Dementia of the Alzheimer's type accounts for what percentage of dementia in the population older than 65 years of age?

a. 10 to 30%
b. 30 to 50%
c. 50 to 70%
d. 70 to 90%
e. Greater than 90%

920. Which of the following is *not* typically associated with dementia?

a. Aphasia
b. Apraxia
c. Agnosia
d. Aprosodia
e. Impaired executive function

921. Which type of dementia typically has the *shortest* duration before death occurs?

a. Alzheimer's disease
b. Vascular dementia
c. Diffuse Lewy body disease
d. Creutzfeldt-Jakob disease
e. Post-concussive dementia

922. Approximately what percentage of the U.S. population greater than 65 years of age suffers from dementia?

a. Five percent
b. 15%
c. 25%
d. 35%
e. 45%

923. Which of the following features is *not* prominent in dementia?

a. Impaired social function
b. Impaired memory
c. Impaired spatial orientation
d. Impaired vision
e. Impaired judgment

924. Pick's disease is *not* typically associated with which of the following?

a. Pathology of the frontal and temporal lobes
b. Loss of social inhibition
c. Personality changes early in the disease
d. Localized cell loss in the hippocampus
e. Memory deficits

925. Stepwise deterioration of cognitive function is typically seen in which of the following?

a. Alzheimer's disease
b. Pick's disease
c. Vascular dementia
d. Dementia pugilistica
e. HIV dementia

926. Which score on the Mini Mental State Examination is considered to be the cutoff for the diagnosis of cognitive dysfunction?

a. 26
b. 23
c. 20
d. 17
e. 14

927. A reversible cause of dementia is

a. Senile dementia of the Alzheimer's type
b. Creutzfeldt-Jakob disease
c. Normal-pressure hydrocephalus
d. Parkinson's disease
e. Vascular dementia

928. Which dementing illness is associated with a gradual decline in memory and social function?

a. Senile dementia of the Alzheimer's type
b. Vascular dementia
c. Creutzfeldt-Jakob disease
d. Pick's disease
e. Pseudodementia of depression

929. A stepwise deterioration is often seen in which of the following types of dementia?

a. Senile dementia of the Alzheimer's type
b. Creutzfeldt-Jakob disease
c. Pick's disease
d. Vascular dementia
e. Pseudodementia of depression

930. The ability to predict suicidal intent may be complicated by which of the following?

a. The physician's emotional reaction toward the patient
b. The physician's knowledge of demographic risk factors
c. Knowledge that a patient has made prior attempts
d. Knowledge of a family history of suicide
e. Knowledge of a personal history of mood disorder

931. The strongest risk factor for suicide listed below is

a. Alcoholism
b. Schizophrenia
c. Major depression
d. Panic disorder
e. Borderline personality disorder

932. Approximately what percentage of completed suicides are thought to be secondary to schizophrenia?

a. Less than one percent
b. Five percent
c. 10%
d. 25%
e. 50%

933. Approximately what percentage of completed suicides are thought to be secondary to major depression?

a. Less than one percent
b. Five percent
c. 10%
d. 25%
e. 50%

934. Approximately what percentage of completed suicides are thought to be secondary to alcoholism and drug dependence?

a. Less than one percent
b. Five percent
c. 10%
d. 25%
e. 50%

935. The chance of suicide is greatest for those who are

a. Married
b. Widowed
c. Separated
d. Divorced
e. Never married

936. Which of the following disorders is *most* closely associated with the risk for suicide?

a. Conversion disorder
b. Post-traumatic stress disorder
c. Panic disorder
d. Obsessive-compulsive disorder
e. Anorexia nervosa

937. Psychiatric hospitalization is *least* often required for patients who

a. Make a violent suicide attempt
b. Take precautions to avoid rescue after a suicide attempt
c. Believe they would die during a suicide attempt
d. Make an impulsive suicide attempt
e. Refuse help after a suicide attempt

938. If one is unsure as to whether a potentially suicidal patient requires psychiatric hospitalization

a. The patient should be admitted
b. The hospital attorney should be consulted
c. The patient's employer should be consulted
d. The patient should be given the option of outpatient follow-up
e. The patient should be sent home with a small amount of medication

939. During the assessment of an anxious, potentially suicidal medical inpatient, it is essential that

a. The patient's employer should be consulted
b. The patient should be protected from harm
c. The patient should be allowed to go outside for a cigarette
d. The patient should be allowed to refuse application of physical restraints
e. The patient should be allowed one phone call

940. Protection of the potentially suicidal patient *rarely* requires

a. Use of physical restraints
b. Prevention of flight from the hospital
c. Avoidance of dangerous objects
d. Presence of a sitter
e. Sedation with a benzodiazepine

941. Suicide assessment *rarely* includes determination as to whether

a. The means of suicide are available
b. There is a plan for suicide
c. There is a precipitant for suicidal ideation
d. The patient has recently read *Final Exit*
e. The patient recently changed his or her will

942. The *least* important question to ask a patient about after a suicide attempt is

a. Did you believe you would die?
b. What was the precipitant?
c. Are you disappointed you survived?
d. What type of health insurance do you have?
e. Do you have realistic plans for the future?

943. Suicide in a general hospital is *least* associated with which of the following conditions?

a. HIV infection
b. Psychosis
c. Chronic renal failure
d. Stroke
e. Pancreatitis

944. Which of the following choices about emotional reactions by physicians to hearing that one's patient has committed suicide is *most* accurate?

a. Emotional reactions are unacceptable.
b. Emotional reactions should be discussed with colleagues.
c. Emotional reactions may include anger.
d. Emotional reactions rarely have an effect on future clinical practice.
e. Emotional reactions are short-lived.

945. The *most* common method of committing suicide is

a. Drug overdose
b. Jumping from a height
c. Use of firearms
d. Hanging
e. Wrist cutting

946. Which of the following statements is *most* accurate about suicide in the United States?

a. Nonwhites are more likely to attempt suicides than whites.
b. Men are more likely to complete suicide than women.
c. More men than women attempt suicide.
d. Suicide rates remain relatively stable during adult life.
e. One of every eight suicide attempts in the elderly is successful.

947. Approximately what percentage of patients with major depression complete suicide?

a. Five percent
b. 10%
c. 15%
d. 20%
e. 25%

948. Death by suicide accounts for

a. Less than 5,000 deaths per year in the United States
b. 20,000 to 40,000 deaths per year in the United States
c. 40,000 to 60,000 deaths per year in the United States
d. 60,000 to 80,000 deaths per year in the United States
e. More than 80,000 deaths per year in the United States

949. The rate of suicide in the general population is

a. 6.7 per 100,000
b. 8.7 per 100,000
c. 10.7 per 100,000
d. 12.7 per 100,000
e. 14.7 per 100,000

950. The *DSM-IV* diagnostic criteria for depression in the medically ill

a. Should be applied to diagnose depression
b. Include disturbance of oxygenation
c. Include nocturnal myoclonus
d. Include disorientation
e. Should be confirmed by a dexamethasone suppression test

951. Post-stroke depression commonly occurs following a stroke in which brain territory?

a. Left frontal area
b. Right posterior area
c. Cerebellum
d. Occipital region
e. Brainstem

952. Right hemisphere lesions commonly result in which of the following?

a. Aprosodias
b. Aphasias
c. SIADH
d. Anisocoria
e. Movement disorders

953. The *most* effective treatment for major depression involves use of which of the following?

a. SSRIs
b. TCAs
c. MAOIs
d. CBT
e. ECT

954. The sedative potency of antidepressants in general correlates with their affinity for which receptors?

a. Dopamine-2 receptors
b. Serotonin receptors
c. Histamine-1 receptors
d. Benzodiazepine receptors
e. Mu receptors

955. Side-effects of TCAs commonly include which of the following?

a. Essential hypertension
b. Conduction system disturbances
c. Cholinergic effects
d. Wolff-Parkinson-White syndrome
e. Congestive heart failure

956. TCA-induced orthostatic hypotension

a. Is rare
b. Often precedes attainment of therapeutic blood levels
c. Can be treated by ingestion of one-inch cubes of cheddar cheese
d. Does not increase in the presence of conduction system disturbance
e. Is more common with nortriptyline than desipramine

957. Which of the following antidepressants would be expected to cause the *least* amount of urinary retention in an elderly man?

a. Nortriptyline
b. Amitriptyline
c. Trazodone
d. Paroxetine
e. Amoxapine

958. Which agent has the greatest activity at the acetylcholine muscarinic receptor?

a. Phenelzine
b. Bupropion
c. Fluoxetine
d. Paroxetine
e. Alprazolam

959. Which of the following electrocardiographic abnormalities is *least* likely to be associated with the use of tricyclic antidepressants?

a. QTc prolongation
b. Development of U waves
c. Prolongation of the PR interval
d. Prolongation of the QRS interval
e. Sinus tachycardia

960. Of the following electrocardiographic abnormalities, the *least* worrisome for a patient about to be started on a tricyclic antidepressant is

a. Left bundle branch block
b. Right bundle branch block
c. Third-degree AV block
d. Atrial fibrillation
e. Ventricular ectopic activity

961. The antidepressant that can be *most* reliably monitored by obtaining serum blood levels is

a. Tranylcypromine
b. Bupropion
c. Alprazolam
d. Nortriptyline
e. Doxepin

962. The side-effect *least* commonly associated with use of methylphenidate in depressed, medically ill adult patients is

a. Anorexia
b. Hypertension
c. Insomnia
d. Tachycardia
e. Cardiac arrhythmias

963. Electrocardiographic abnormalities associated with lithium use in the medically ill include each of the following choices *except*

a. First-degree AV block
b. Development of U waves
c. T-wave flattening
d. Non-specific ST and T-wave changes
e. Prolongation of the QRS interval

964. Symptoms of dysthymia include each of the following *except*

a. Disturbed appetite
b. Disturbed sleep patterns
c. Fatigue
d. Mood lability
e. Disturbed concentration ability

965. Indications for electroconvulsive therapy include each of the following *except*

a. Delusional depression
b. Mania
c. Schizophrenia
d. Catatonia
e. Hypochondriasis

966. The complication *least* likely to be associated with catatonic syndromes is

a. Decubitus ulcers
b. Pneumonia
c. Seizures
d. Limb contractures
e. Pulmonary emboli

967. Which of the following conditions is *not* an indication for ECT?

a. Catatonia
b. Schizophrenia
c. Neuroleptic malignant syndrome
d. Tardive dyskinesia
e. Psychotic depression

968. Which of the following is *not* an adverse effect of ECT?

a. Complex partial seizures
b. Amnesia
c. Confusion
d. Catatonia
e. Sinus arrest

969. Which of the following statements about ECT is *false?*

a. Cardiac arrhythmia is a relative contraindication for ECT.
b. Having an AV malformation is an absolute contraindication for ECT.
c. ECT is relatively safe 30 to 60 days after a cerebral infarction.
d. An ejection fraction below 20% is an absolute contraindication for ECT.
e. ECT has a higher rate of response than antidepressants for depression.

970. Which drug is typically *not* used just before or during ECT?

a. Labetalol
b. Esmolol
c. Methohexital
d. Diazepam
e. Succinylcholine

971. What is the mortality rate associated with ECT?

a. 0.0003%
b. 0.03%
c. 0.3%
d. One percent
e. Three percent

972. Which of the following statements about maintenance ECT is *true?*

a. It is always the first choice after a good response to an initial trial of ECT.
b. It is less efficacious than MAOIs in preventing relapse.
c. It can be combined with psychotropic medication.
d. It is not likely to prevent a relapse.
e. It is rarely recommended.

973. Seizure activity in which brain structure is thought to be essential for the efficacy of ECT?

a. The frontal lobe
b. The temporal lobe
c. The hypothalamus
d. The pituitary gland
e. The thalamus

974. Which of the following statements about the stimulus used for seizure induction during ECT is *true*?

a. Unilateral sine-wave stimulus is the preferred technique.
b. Bilateral brief-pulse wave stimulus is not recommended.
c. Sine-wave stimuli cause less amnesia than brief-pulse wave stimuli.
d. Patients should always be treated with bilateral stimuli.
e. High centro-parietal and fronto-temporal locations are the preferred positions for bilateral stimulation.

975. What percentage of patients experience short-term remission of depressive symptoms after ECT?

a. 20%
b. 40%
c. 60%
d. 80%
e. 100%

976. Relapse into depression within the first year after a single course, encompassing six to eight sessions, of ECT is seen in approximately what percentage of depressed patients?

a. Zero percent
b. 20%
c. 50%
d. 80%
e. 100%

977. Which of the following is an *absolute contraindication* to ECT?

a. Congestive heart failure
b. Recent myocardial infarction
c. Hypertension
d. Meningioma
e. None of the above

978. Which of the following statements concerning the period after the seizure induced by ECT is *false?*

a. Parasympathetic tone remains strong.
b. Transient bradycardia occurs.
c. Cardiac output decreases abruptly.
d. Transient hypotension occurs.
e. Circulating catecholamine levels rise.

979. For patients with depression and coronary artery disease undergoing ECT, which class of short-acting medication is often administered to reduce cardiac complications?

a. Benzodiazepines
b. Muscle relaxants
c. Beta-blockers
d. Barbiturates
e. Anticholinergics

980. Fluent aphasias are associated with lesions in which of the following brain areas?

a. Papez's circuit
b. Wernicke's area
c. Broca's area
d. The brainstem
e. The nucleus accumbens

981. Which of the following brain regions is considered to be part of the limbic system?

a. The superior colliculus
b. The hypothalamus
c. The lateral geniculate nucleus
d. The cerebellum
e. The pituitary gland

982. Who coined the term *limbic system?*

a. Paul Broca
b. James Papez
c. Paul MacLean
d. Walle Nauta
e. George Murray

983. Which brain structure is *not* part of the language circuit?

a. Wernicke's area
b. The superior temporal gyrus
c. The arcuate fasciculus
d. Broca's area
e. The superior frontal gyrus

984. Schizophrenia has been associated with pathology in which of the following brain areas?

a. The spinal cord
b. The occipital cortex
c. The lateral geniculate nucleus
d. The medial dorsal thalamic nucleus
e. The medial geniculate nucleus

985. Which of the following brain regions is *not* part of the limbic system?

a. The hypothalamus
b. The hippocampus
c. The amygdala
d. The thalamus
e. The parietal cortex

986. Which brain region is *not* part of the frontal lobe?

a. The cingulate cortex
b. The supplementary motor area
c. The premotor cortex
d. The motor cortex
e. The insula

987. Which of the following is *not* typically seen after a stroke in the left hemisphere?

a. Depression
b. Aphasia
c. Aprosodia
d. Delirium
e. Eye deviation to the left

988. Which brain region has progressed the *most* throughout phylogeny?

a. The frontal lobe
b. The temporal lobe
c. The parietal lobe
d. The occipital lobe
e. The thalamus

989. Which abnormality is *not* associated with diffuse frontal lobe dysfunction?

a. The palmomental reflex
b. The snout reflex
c. The Babinski sign
d. The Svotchec sign
e. A lack of habituation to glabellar tapping

990. Lesions in which brain area are usually associated with aprosodias?

a. The occipital lobes
b. The cerebellum
c. The right hemisphere
d. The left hemisphere
e. The hypothalamus

991. Lesions in which brain area are usually associated with aphasias?

a. The occipital lobes
b. The cerebellum
c. The right hemisphere
d. The left hemisphere
e. The hypothalamus

992. Lesions in which brain area are usually associated with expressive aphasias?

a. Wernicke's area
b. Broca's area
c. Papez's circuit
d. The substantia nigra
e. The nucleus accumbens

993. Lesions in which brain area are usually associated with receptive aphasias?

a. Wernicke's area
b. Broca's area
c. Papez's circuit
d. The substantia nigra
e. The nucleus accumbens

994. Lesions in which brain area are usually associated with fluent aphasias?

a. Wernicke's area
b. Broca's area
c. Papez's circuit
d. The substantia nigra
e. The nucleus accumbens

995. Lesions in which brain area are usually associated with nonfluent aphasias?

a. Wernicke's area
b. Broca's area
c. Papez's circuit
d. The substantia nigra
e. The nucleus accumbens

996. Which of the following conditions is thought to be characterized by defective regulation of the transport of calcium ions by the sarcoplastic reticulum?

a. Serotonin syndrome
b. Catatonia
c. Malignant hyperthermia
d. Neuroleptic malignant syndrome
e. Tetanus

997. Which of the following is *not* a typical clinical feature of neuroleptic malignant syndrome (NMS)?

a. CPK elevation
b. Fever
c. Leukocytosis
d. Mydriasis
e. Autonomic dysfunction

998. The pathophysiology of NMS is thought to involve each of the following *except*

a. Blockade of central dopamine receptors
b. Blockade of peripheral dopamine receptors in smooth muscle
c. Blockade of peripheral serotonin receptors
d. Blockade of post-ganglionic sympathetic neurons
e. Blockade of dopamine receptors in the hypothalamus and basal ganglia

999. Which of the following statements is *not* true about malignant hyperthermia (MH)?

a. There is often a temporal relationship to the administration of halogenated inhalation anesthetics.
b. There is often a temporal relationship to the administration of succinylcholine.
c. There is often a family history of malignant hyperthermia.
d. There is often a positive response to treatment with IV bromocriptine.
e. There is often a positive response to treatment with IV dantrolene.

1000. Which of the following is *not* a feature of anticholinergic delirium?

a. A positive response to IV physostigmine
b. Tachycardia
c. Fever
d. Diaphoresis
e. Mydriasis

Answers

1. The answer is c. *DSM-IV* criteria for major depressive disorder include depressed mood (but in children and adolescents it may be irritable mood) or markedly diminished interest or pleasure in almost all activities for two or more weeks, and five or more of the following symptoms: depressed mood; loss of interest or pleasure; significant weight loss or gain, or decreased or increased appetite; insomnia or hypersomnia; psychomotor agitation or retardation; feelings of worthlessness or excessive or inappropriate guilt; fatigue or loss of energy; diminished ability to concentrate; recurrent thoughts of death or suicide. Panic attacks often co-exist with depressive disorders but are not a diagnostic feature of major depression. (1.13.c.g.d.m.a.14)

2. The answer is c. Less than 50% of patients with MDD receive treatment for their condition. Barriers (e.g., visits with physicians are often too short to allow for attention to the variety of problems faced by patients) exist to the prompt recognition of the syndrome, which leads to inadequate treatment of depression. (2.13.60.c.g.d.t.m.a.14)

3. The answer is e. *DSM-IV* criteria for dysthymic disorder include depressed mood (or irritable mood in children and adolescents) for at least one year for most of the day, for more days than not, for at least two years, and the presence, when depressed, of at least two of the following: poor appetite or overeating, insomnia or hypersomnia, low energy or fatigue, low self-esteem, poor concentration, or feelings of hopelessness. Recurrent thoughts of death or suicide are criteria for major depressive disorder, not dysthymia. (3.13.c.g.d.m.a.14)

4. The answer is b. SSRIs are typically not very anticholinergic, so anticholinergic symptoms (e.g., constipation and dry mouth) are relatively infrequent with their usage. (4.31.c.p.t.m.a.14)

5. The answer is d. Orthostatic hypotension is not due to muscarinic receptor blockade; instead it is due to α_1-adrenergic receptor blockade. (5.31.c.p.t.m.a.14)

6. The answer is c. Histamine H_1 receptor blockade causes sedation, increased appetite, weight gain, hypotension, and potentiation of central depressant drugs. (6.31.c.p.t.m.a.14)

7. The answer is d. Paroxetine is a selective serotonin reuptake inhibitor (SSRI). (7.31.c.p.t.m.a.14)

8. The answer is c. Amoxapine, doxepin, and trimipramine are tricyclic antidepressants (TCAs), while venlafaxine is a selective serotonin reuptake inhibitor (SSRI). (8.31.c.p.t.m.a.14)

9. The answer is a. Since the risk of seizures in bupropion-treated patients was noted to be higher in patients with bulimia than in non-eating-disordered patients, its use in eating-disordered patients is contraindicated. (9.21.31.c.p.t.m.a.14)

10. The answer is d. Bupropion lacks significant anticholinergic, antihistaminic, and anti-α_1-adrenergic effects, so that side effects such as blurred vision, urinary retention, weight gain, sedation, and orthostatic hypotension are relatively infrequent with this antidepressant. (10.31.c.p.t.m.a.14)

11. The answer is b. Mirtazapine has significant histamine H_1 receptor blocking activity, which accounts for its ability to cause sedation, increased appetite, and weight gain. (11.31.c.p.t.m.a.14)

12. The answer is c. Phenelzine and other MAOIs are associated with a risk of lethal hypertensive crisis related to interactions with foods containing tyramine and with sympathomimetic drugs. (12.31.c.p.t.m.a.14)

13. The answer is e. Increased intracranial pressure, coronary artery disease, digitalis toxicity, and intracranial lesions are relative, but not absolute, contraindications to the use of ECT. (13.43.c.g.t.m.a.14)

14. The answer is d. Less than 50% of depressed patients typically show a robust response to treatment, with a substantial proportion of patients showing only a partial but significant improvement. Many patients take five to eight weeks to show significant improvement; therefore, at least six weeks of treatment with a given antidepressant is indicated. A combination of antidepressants and antianxiety drugs, to address nervousness and agitation, is relatively common in depression. Clinicians tend to use drugs with the lowest side-effect burden, as the likelihood of continuing antidepressant treatment is greater if an agent is well tolerated. (14.31.c.p.t.m.a.14)

15. The answer is a. The risk of relapse after antidepressant withdrawal only abates after at least four months of a sustained response to treatment. (15.13.31.c.g.p.t.m.a.14)

16. The answer is c. Survival of a premeditated attempt is associated with a higher risk of making another attempt. (16.38.c.g.d.m.a.15)

17. The answer is c. Suicide is the third-leading cause of death in those between the ages of 15 and 24 years. (17.38.63.c.g.d.m.a.15)

18. The answer is d. Those who are widowed have a greater risk than those who are divorced, or those who are married. (18.38.63.c.g.d.m.a.15)

19. The answer is a. Medication may be advisable for agitation that jeopardizes the safety of the patient or the staff. Failure to cooperate, in and of itself, is not an indication for pharmacotherapy. (19.38.c.g.d.t.m.a.15)

20. The answer is e. Disorientation is a feature of delirium and other organic brain syndromes, not of anxiety. (20.15.c.g.d.m.a.16)

21. The answer is b. The locus coeruleus is a storehouse of noradrenergic innervation; it is associated with panic when stimulated. (21.15.g.d.m.a.16)

22. The answer is c. Agents that block locus coeruleus firing and norepinephrine output, e.g., antidepressants and high-potency benzodiazepines, decrease panic attacks. (22.15.g.p.d.a.16)

23. The answer is d. Anxiety is particularly common in the general medical setting; it is one of the most common chief complaints for people seeking care from a primary care physician, occurring in 10% of patients. (23.15.c.g.d.m.a.16)

24. The answer is e. However, 20 to 40% of patients with irritable bowel syndrome have PD, and irritable bowel symptoms are troubling for many patients with PD. (24.15.c.g.d.m.a.16)

25. The answer is e. Chest pain is common in patients with panic disorder (PD). PD occurs in 10 to 20% of patients who present to emergency rooms with chest pain. The concurrence of pain and chest pain results in increased usage of emergency rooms and intensive care facilities and accounts for an increase in cardiac work-ups. (25.15.45.c.g.d.m.a.16)

26. The answer is c. Onset of symptoms after the age of 35, lack of a personal or family history of an anxiety disorder, lack of avoidance behavior, and a poor response to anti-panic agents supports an organic anxiety disorder, but a history of spontaneous anxiety is more suggestive of a primary anxiety disorder. (26.15.c.g.d.m.a.16)

27. The answer is e. Beta-adrenergic agonists, not beta-blockers, are associated with anxiety symptoms. However, beta-blockers have been associated with psychiatric symptoms (confusion, psychosis, agitation, anxiety, depression) in patients taking propranolol, metoprolol, and other beta-blockers for medical indications. (27.9.15.37.c.g.p.t.m.a.16)

28. The answer is c. Diabetes (with hypoglycemic episodes), hyperthyroidism, complex partial seizures, and COPD all contribute to anxiety symptoms. (28.9.15.c.g.d.m.a.16)

29. The answer is a. Typically, panic disorder begins in the second or third decade of life, though many patients first experience anxiety difficulties in childhood. (29.15.g.d.m.a.16)

30. The answer is b. While the other disorders cited are associated with anxiety, they do not have discrete episodes that peak in intensity in 10 minutes. (30.15.g.d.m.a.16)

31. The answer is a. (31.15.g.d.m.a.16)

32. The answer is d. The other conditions listed, while associated with anxiety symptoms, do not involve exposure to the threat of death or injury. (32.15.16.g.d.m.a.16)

33. The answer is d. While the tricyclic antidepressants (TCAs) are effective for panic disorder and generalized anxiety disorder, and less so for social phobia, with the exception of clomipramine, TCAs are largely ineffective for obsessive-compulsive disorder (OCD). Clomipramine is primarily a serotonin uptake inhibitor, which may account for its efficacy in the treatment of OCD. Its major metabolite is a noradrenergic uptake blocker. (33.15.29.31.g.p.t.m.a.16)

34. The answer is c. Oxazepam, with a slow onset of action, has a half-life of 5 to 15 hours. Clonazepam, with an intermediate onset of action, has a half-life of 15 to 50 hours. Clorazepate, with a rapid onset of action, has a half-life of 30 to 200 hours. Alprazolam, with an intermediate to fast onset of action, has a half-life of 12 to 15 hours. Lorazepam, with an intermediate onset of action, has a half-life of 10 to 20 hours. Dose equivalents are: oxazepam, 15 mg; clonazepam, 0.25 mg; clorazepate, 7.5 mg; alprazolam, 0.5 mg; and lorazepam, 1 mg. (34.15.29.c.g.p.t.m.a.16)

35. The answer is a. Oxazepam lacks significant metabolites and requires only glucuronidation by the liver. (35.15.29.c.g.p.t.m.a.16)

36. The answer is b. Half-lives of the listed medications are: alprazolam, 12 to 15 hours; clorazepate, 30 to 200 hours; chlordiazepoxide, 5 to 30 hours; lorazepam, 10 to 20 hours; and oxazepam, 5 to 15 hours. (36.15.29.c.g.p.t.m.a.16)

37. The answer is d. As a rule, benzodiazepines elevate rather than reduce the seizure threshold. This is one of the reasons that many patients undergoing electroconvulsive therapy (ECT) have their benzodiazepines held prior to ECT. (37.15.29.c.g.p.t.m.a.16)

38. The answer is d. Increased gastrointestinal motility, rather than constipation, is more likely to be associated with withdrawal from benzodiazepines. (38.15.29.c.g.p.t.m.a.16)

39. The answer is c. Each of the other choices is a common response to stress. (39.15.45.56.57.c.g.d.m.a.11)

40. The answer is d. Dilated pupils, not constricted (or miotic) pupils, are found in response to stress or anxiety. (40.15.c.g.d.m.a.11)

41. The answer is b. Projection, a primitive psychological defense, is not taught as a technique to deal with stress reactions. (41.15.56.57.g.t.m.a.11)

42. The answer is a. Daily hassles, self-doubt, a perceived lack of support from family or friends, down-sizing at work, and an overload of responsibilities can also contribute to stress reactions. Benzodiazepine withdrawal results in anxiety symptoms but not a stress response. (42.15.29.56.57.d.m.a.11)

43. The answer is d. Payment method for services does not in general help one's understanding of chronic stress, although it may be correlated with other indicators of social connectedness. (43.15.56.57.g.d.m.a.11)

44. The answer is a. Stress causes a lowering of skin temperature. (44.15.56.57.g.d.m.a.11)

45. The answer is e. While cognitive restructuring is a technique to decrease stress, it is not in and of itself a relaxation-training exercise. (45.15.56.57.69.g.t.m.a.11)

46. The answer is b. Incredibly, 50% of trauma beds are filled with patients injured while under the influence of alcohol. (46.10.63.c.g.d.m.a.52)

47. The answer is a. However, alcohol abuse must be diagnosed if the patient has met criteria for alcohol dependence. (47.10.c.g.d.m.a.52)

48. The answer is c. (48.10.63.c.g.d.m.a.52)

49. The answer is b. (49.10.63.c.g.d.m.a.52)

50. The answer is e. Cutting down, being annoyed, feeling guilty, and having an eye-opener are screening criteria for the CAGE questionnaire. While many alcoholics believe it is easy to stop drinking, that statement is not one of the CAGE criteria. (50.10.61.c.g.d.m.a.52)

51. The answer is c. (51.9.10.c.g.d.m.a.52)

52. The answer is c. Two or more positive responses on the CAGE questionnaire correlate with significant alcohol-related problems. (52.10.61.c. g.d.m.a.52)

53. The answer is e. More than 60% are either depressed or dysthymic during the early months of sobriety. (53.10.c.g.d.m.a.52)

54. The answer is b. Long-lasting benzodiazepines provide a "smoother ride" and are generally preferred for detoxification to prevent withdrawal symptoms. (54.10.c.g.p.t.m.a.52)

55. The answer is c. Lorazepam is preferred because it is relatively short-lasting and requires only glucouronidation, and not oxidative metabolism by the liver. (55.10.29.c.g.p.t.m.a.52)

56. The answer is b. Naltrexone is an opiate antagonist. (56.11.c.g.p.t.m. a.52)

57. The answer is e. Liver function needs to be monitored because disulfiram can cause hepatitis. (57.11.c.g.p.t.m.a.52)

58. The answer is d. The prevalence of migraines in females is thought to be 20%. (58.63.75.c.g.d.m.a.26)

59. The answer is a. A family history of cluster headaches is rarely found. (59.63.75.c.g.d.m.a.26)

60. The answer is a. Migraines are usually unilateral, in the frontotemporal area. (60.75.c.g.d.m.a.26)

61. The answer is c. Cluster headaches come on quickly and peak in 5 to 10 minutes. (61.75.c.g.d.m.a.26)

62. The answer is true. (62.75.c.g.d.f.a.26)

63. The answer is true. (63.75.c.g.d.f.a.26)

64. The answer is false. (64.75.c.g.d.f.a.26)

65. The answer is true. (65.75.c.g.d.f.a.26)

66. The answer is false. (66.75.c.g.d.f.a.26)

67. The answer is true. (67.75.c.g.d.f.a.26)

68. The answer is false. (68.75.c.g.d.f.a.26)

69. The answer is true. (69.75.c.g.d.f.a.26)

70. The answer is true. (70.75.c.g.d.f.a.26)

71. The answer is true. (71.75.c.g.d.f.a.26)

72. The answer is true. (72.75.c.g.d.f.a.26)

73. The answer is true. (73.75.c.g.d.f.a.26)

74. The answer is e. Propranolol is used for prophylaxis, not for acute treatment. (74.75.c.g.p.t.m.a.26)

75. The answer is d. Sumatriptan is used for acute treatment only. (75.75.c.g.p.t.m.a.26)

76. The answer is e. Propranolol is used for migraine prophylaxis, not for acute treatment of cluster headaches. (76.75.c.g.p.t.m.a.26)

77. The answer is d. Restless legs syndrome is often thought of as a pre-sleep phenomenon, causing dyssomnia; it is not a parasomnia. (77.22.c.g.d.m.a.27)

78. The answer is d. The immediate onset of REM sleep is characteristic of narcolepsy, not of prolonged sleep latency. (78.22.c.g.d.m.a.27)

79. The answer is d. Core temperature may be recorded, but skin temperature is not. (79.22.c.g.d.m.a.27)

80. The answer is e. Bupropion, with an amphetamine-like structure, tends to be activating, not sedating. (80.22.31.c.g.p.t.m.a.27)

81. The answer is d. Hypersomnia may occur during conversations or while performing potentially hazardous activities. (81.22.c.g.d.m.a.27)

82. The answer is d. All of the other treatments mentioned target improved function in the upper airways that minimize obstruction. (82.22.c.g.t.m.a.27)

83. The answer is c. While the presence of the other conditions does not make one immune to snoring, obstructive sleep apnea commonly leads to loud snoring. (83.22.c.g.d.m.a.27)

84. The answer is e. Five or more episodes of apnea or hypopnea per hour of sleep are required for the diagnosis to be made. (84.22.c.g.d.m.a.27)

85. The answer is a. Sleepwalking, a parasomnia, is not one of the diagnostic features of narcolepsy. (85.22.c.g.d.m.a.27)

86. The answer is d. (86.22.c.g.d.m.a.27)

87. The answer is c. (87.22.c.g.d.m.a.27)

88. The answer is b. (88.22.c.g.d.m.a.27)

89. The answer is a. (89.22.c.g.d.m.a.27)

90. The answer is e. (90.22.c.g.d.m.a.27)

91. The answer is e. (91.22.c.g.d.m.a.27)

92. The answer is a. (92.22.c.g.d.m.a.27)

93. The answer is d. (93.22.c.g.d.m.a.27)

94. The answer is b. (94.22.c.g.d.m.a.27)

95. The answer is c. (95.22.c.g.d.m.a.27)

96. The answer is e. Craniopharyngiomas are not typically associated with dizziness as they are not in proximity to structures related to equilibrium. (96.37.c.g.d.m.a.28)

97. The answer is e. Labyrinthitis is a peripheral, not a central, cause of vertigo. (97.37.c.g.d.m.a.28)

98. The answer is true. (98.37.c.g.d.f.a.28)

99. The answer is true. (99.37.c.g.d.f.a.28)

100. The answer is false. While the syndrome is characterized by attacks of severe vertigo and vomiting, tinnitus, and fluctuating hearing loss, consciousness is not lost. (100.37.c.g.d.f.a.28)

101. The answer is d. Multiple sclerosis is a central, not a systemic, cause of vertigo. (101.37.c.g.d.m.a.28)

102. The answer is e. Actually, fatigue is one of the most common complaints (unrelated to age), and it is more common in women than among men. (102.17.c.g.d.m.a.34)

103. The answer is d. While anemia may cause fatigue, an isolated decrease in platelets is not associated with fatigue. (103.17.c.g.d.m.a.34)

104. The answer is b. Diagnoses that involve simulation or feigning disease include malingering and factitious disorder. They can be distinguished by the reason for the deception. With malingering there is a clear-cut secondary gain, and with factitious disorder the goal is to become a patient. (104.17.c.g.d.m.a.29)

105. The answer is a. While *la belle indifférence* can be seen in conversion disorder, right parietal lesions may involve hemi-neglect and indifference. (105.17.c.g.d.m.a.29)

106. The answer is e. Pimozide, a neuroleptic used to treat monosymptomatic hypochondriacal psychosis, is not a standard treatment for hypochondriasis, and it rarely leads to relief of hypochondriacal symptoms. (106.17.c.g.d.m.a.29)

107. The answer is e. Temporal lobe epilepsy is not a systemic disorder, though it may result in isolated or recurrent neurologic complaints. (107.17.c.g.d.m.a.29)

108. The answer is true. (108.15.17.c.g.d.f.a.29)

109. The answer is true. (109.17.c.g.d.f.a.29)

110. The answer is false. Sixty-five percent of patients with hypochondriasis have concurrent personality disorder, and 72% of patients with somatization disorder have concurrent personality disorder. (110.17.63.c.g.d.f.a.29)

111. The answer is false. These are features of hypochondriasis. (111.17.c.g.d.f.a.29)

112. The answer is false. These are features of somatization disorder. (112.17.c.g.d.f.a.29)

113. The answer is c. These are not culturally-sanctioned responses. (113.17.c.g.d.m.a.29)

114. The answer is a. Intentionally feigned symptoms are not part of somatization disorder. (114.17.c.g.d.m.a.29)

115. The answer is e. Objective complaints rather than subjective complaints should be investigated. (115.17.c.g.t.m.a.29)

116. The answer is e. (116.9.17.c.g.d.m.a.35)

117. The answer is d. (117.9.17.c.g.d.m.a.35)

118. The answer is a. Symptoms of chronic fatigue syndrome overlap those of many psychiatric and medical diagnoses including fibromyalgia, Epstein-Barr syndrome, multiple allergy syndrome, and multiple chemical sensitivity syndrome. (118.9.17.c.g.d.m.a.35)

119. The answer is e. Since major depression is often diagnosed in those with chronic fatigue syndrome, it should be sought out and treated aggressively to minimize disability and dysfunction. (119.9.17.c.g.t.m.a.35)

120. The answer is e. Such diagnostic tests used by clinical ecologists have not been validated. (120.17.c.g.t.m.a.36)

121. The answer is d. Although the physical exam of the patient is typically normal, it should be done and should focus on the examination of the skin, the eyes, and the oral pharynx for evidence of inflammation. Examination of the liver, spleen, and for the presence of lymph nodes should also be performed. (121.17.c.g.d.m.a.36)

122. The answer is e. IBS is a motor disorder of the bowel that may lead to passage of the stool mucus but not to bleeding. (122.17.c.g.d.m.a.37)

123. The answer is e. Among patients with IBS, there is an association between a history of sexual or physical abuse and seeking care for symptoms. (123.17.c.g.d.m.a.37)

124. The answer is e. Even obsessive-compulsive disorder (OCD) is more prevalent than conversion disorder; many clinicians refer to IBS patients as having bowel obsession. (124.17.c.g.d.m.a.37)

125. The answer is d. Payment for the evaluation comes from the party requesting the evaluation. (125.40.g.t.m.a.63)

126. The answer is e. Just the opposite of the statement in **e** is correct. (126.40.g.t.m.a.63)

127. The answer is true. (127.40.g.d.f.a.63)

128. The answer is true. (128.40.g.d.f.a.63)

129. The answer is false. Rarely are these details necessary in disability reports. Even though confidentiality is limited, information should be shared on a need-to-know basis, and a note stating that the limits of confidentiality were discussed with the patient should be included. (129.40.g.t.f.a.63)

130. The answer is true. (130.40.g.t.f.a.63)

131. The answer is false. These tests can be especially helpful. (131.40.g.d.f.a.63)

132. The answer is true. (132.40.g.t.f.a.63)

133. The answer is false. This is a key function of the report. (133.40. g.t.f.a.63)

134. The answer is d. Denial represents a normal response to acute stress. (134.45.c.g.d.m.a.62)

135. The answer is true. (135.45.c.g.d.f.a.62)

136. The answer is false. Right-sided parietal lesions and sometimes subcortical lesions can cause neglect of hemiplegic limbs, usually on the left side of the body. (136.37.44.45.72.c.g.d.f.a.62)

137. The answer is true. This syndrome is often termed Anton's syndrome. (137.37.45.72.c.g.d.f.a.62)

138. The answer is e. Benzodiazepines may relieve anxiety, which may then allow the patient to consider evaluation and treatment. However, the physician should respect the patient's decision to take a less active role in medical management. (138.45.c.g.t.m.a.62)

139. The answer is false. Symptoms are under-reported, and patients and family members blame them on advancing age. (139.42.c.g.d.f.a.49)

140. The answer is true. (140.42.c.g.d.f.a.49)

141. The answer is true. (141.42.c.g.d.f.a.49)

142. The answer is true. (142.42.c.g.d.f.a.49)

143. The answer is true. (143.42.c.g.d.f.a.49)

144. The answer is true. (144.42.c.g.d.f.a.49)

145. The answer is e. Shopping is an independent activity of daily living, not a basic activity of daily living. (145.42.c.g.d.m.a.49)

146. The answer is true. If cognitive impairment is present, combining the GDS with the Mini Mental State Examination may be helpful. (146.42. c.g.d.f.a.49)

147. The answer is false. Frontal lobe function is inadequately assessed by means of the MMSE. (147.2.8.42.61.72.c.g.d.f.a.49)

148. The answer is false. It primarily tests for attention and calculation ability. (148.42.61.72.82.c.g.d.f.a.49)

149. The answer is b. Adjustment reactions may, however, be more commonplace as patients adapt to potentially life-threatening illness. (149.13. 44.45.63.c.g.d.m.a.38)

150. The answer is d. Variable moods in the first few months after the diagnosis of cancer is reached can be part of a normal response. (150.44. 45.c.g.d.m.a.38)

151. The answer is d. IL-2 commonly causes delirium, but not just lethargy. (151.36.45.c.g.p.d.m.a.38)

152. The answer is d. The others are not hormonal agents, though they are anti-cancer drugs. Procarbazine and 5-fluouricil are chemotherapeutic agents, while interferon and interleukin-2 (IL-2) are biologicals. (152.45.c. g.p.t.m.a.38)

153. The answer is e. Affective, behavioral, and cognitive symptoms are common with corticosteroids. As the dose of corticosteroids increases, so does the frequency of side effects. (153.36.c.g.p.t.m.a.38)

154. The answer is c. Not a dopamine blocker, unlike the other agents listed, aminoglutethimide may cause rash, malaise, and fatigue, but not akathisia. (154.30.36.c.g.p.t.m.a.38)

155. The answer is c. Hypocalcemia, not hypercalcemia, is associated with tetany. (155.36.c.g.p.t.m.a.38)

156. The answer is d. Psychological reactions to the diagnosis of cancer include anxiety and depression but do not result in a syndrome of delirium. (156.6.9.44.45.c.g.p.d.m.a.38)

157. The answer is d. The syndrome is associated with limbic encephalitis but not with metastatic lesions per se in the cerebrum. (157.6.9.44.c.g. d.m.a.38)

158. The answer is a. While sumatriptan can reduce nausea and vomiting associated with migraine headaches, it is not generally used to treat post-chemotherapy nausea and vomiting. (158.36.44.c.g.p.t.m.a.38)

159. The answer is d. Ondansetron and granisetron are both $5HT_3$ antagonists. (159.28.36.44.c.g.p.t.m.a.38)

160. The answer is b. Metoclopramide is both a cholinergic and a dopamine antagonist. (160.28.36.44.c.g.p.t.m.a.38)

161. The answer is e. Palliative care is not euthanasia. The goal of palliative care is to do whatever it takes to alleviate suffering. (161.45.49.c.g. t.m.a.51)

162. The answer is true. (162.45.49.c.g.t.f.a.51)

163. The answer is true. (163.45.49.c.g.t.f.a.51)

164. The answer is true. (164.45.49.c.g.t.f.a.51)

165. The answer is false. Typically in patients with terminal illness, an expected survival of less than six months is required to be eligible for hospice care. (165.45.49.c.g.t.f.a.51)

166. The answer is false. The amount and detail provided to a patient should be consonant with the patient's response to general questions and his or her capacity to understand and deal with information. (166.45.49. c.g.t.f.a.51)

167. The answer is false. Indeed, a shift to palliative care focuses treatment away from aggressive treatment aimed at cure and toward the relief of suffering. (167.44.45.49.c.g.t.f.a.51)

168. The answer is false. Food and drink should be allowed ad lib for comfort. (168.44.45.49.c.g.t.f.a.51)

169. The answer is true. (169.44.45.49.c.g.d.f.a.51)

170. The answer is true. (170.44.45.49.c.g.d.f.a.51)

171. The answer is true. Similarly, mental disorders are appropriately left untreated in the setting of terminal illness when they do not cause substantial suffering or when the treatment might place the patient at risk for more suffering. (171.44.45.49.c.g.t.f.a.51)

172. The answer is false. Just the opposite. They are under-recognized and under-treated. Recognition may be hindered by the clinician's limited experience in diagnosing mental disorders in the setting of serious physical illness, by the difficulty of interpreting clinical information in the setting of premorbid psychiatric disorders, and by concerns about stigmatization if a diagnosis of a mental disorder is made. (172.44.45.49.c.g.d.f.a.51)

173. The answer is false. While worry, fearfulness, discouragement, and sadness are seen at least transiently in many, if not all, patients with terminal illness, manifestations of mental disorders cause substantial suffering. (173.44.45.49.c.g.d.f.a.51)

174. The answer is false. Estimates vary, but as many as 77% of patients with terminal illness may suffer from clinically significant depression. (174.13.44.45.49.63.c.g.d.f.a.51)

175. The answer is false. As many as 85% of all patients may develop delirium near the end of life. (175.6.44.45.63.c.g.d.f.a.51)

176. The answer is d. Both dextroamphetamine and methylphenidate have a low potential for abuse in this patient population and are often the drugs of choice for depressive symptoms in patients with terminal illness. (176.34.44.c.g.p.t.m.a.51)

177. The answer is d. When delivering bad news, it is best to be succinct. In this highly stressful situation, brevity and technical simplicity are useful for communication to be efficient. (177.44.45.49.c.g.t.m.a.75)

178. The answer is true. The physician may be able to offer reassurance to the patient that pain can and will be attacked throughout the illness. (178.44.45.49.c.g.t.f.a.75)

179. The answer is false. At no time is trust more important between a physician and a patient and family than in the presence of a severe illness or death. (179.44.45.49.c.g.t.f.a.75)

180. The answer is true. A parent may have difficulty relating to a child. This is especially problematic after the death of a parent. (180.44.45.49.c.g.t.f.a.75)

181. The answer is true. (181.44.45.49.c.g.t.f.a.75)

182. The answer is true. (182.44.45.49.c.g.t.f.a.75)

183. The answer is false. While the loss of a pregnancy is less devastating than the death of a living child, the intensity of grief often is surprisingly severe. Physicians can help mitigate the impact of those who urge grieving parents to get over their loss quickly. (183.44.45.49.c.g.t.f.a.75)

184. The answer is true. (184.45.c.g.t.f.a.75)

185. The answer is a. Most patients in this situation do not worry about the physician's theories of attribution regarding the illness. (185.44.45.49. c.g.t.m.a.75)

186. The answer is d. There may be a circumstance where catastrophic loss is experienced—for example, when identification with the patient and his or her illness is faced—but the other feelings listed are generally more common. (186.44.45.49.c.g.t.m.a.75)

187. The answer is true. (187.39.44.49.c.g.t.f.a.70)

188. The answer is false. In physician-assisted suicide, the physician provides the sufficient means of death to the patient who performs the final act. The physician who administers a lethal dose of medication to a patient with the intent to end that patient's life is performing euthanasia or committing murder. (188.39.44.49.c.g.t.f.a.70)

189. The answer is true. (189.39.44.49.c.g.t.f.a.70)

190. The answer is true. (190.39.44.49.c.g.t.f.a.70)

191. The answer is true. Competency is a legal concept. The physician in effect assesses whether the patient has capacity, and this lays the groundwork for determination of the patient's competency by a court of law. (191.39.44.c.g.d.f.a.70)

192. The answer is true. (192.44.49.c.g.t.f.a.70)

193. The answer is true. (193.39.44.49.c.g.d.f.a.70)

194. The answer is false. The decisions of a health care proxy come into play when the patient no longer has the capacity to make treatment decisions. (194.39.44.49.c.g.t.f.a.70)

195. The answer is false. While not required, this is a strategy that provides help with continued decision-making. (195.39.44.49.c.g.t.f.a.70)

196. The answer is true. (196.39.44.49.c.g.t.f.a.70)

197. The answer is true. A trial court may decide that a patient would die in a short period of time with or without treatment. A physician would not be negligent in not administering that treatment. (197.39.44.49.c.g.t.f.a.70)

198. The answer is true. (198.39.44.49.c.g.t.f.a.70)

199. The answer is false. Good documentation is important. However, documentation is not required to protect against future changes in decisions. (199.39.44.49.c.g.t.f.a.70)

200. The answer is c. A competent patient's preferences should be adhered to. The view of the health care proxy comes into question later in the course of illness. (200.39.44.49.c.g.t.m.a.70)

201. The answer is c. Grief is a variable but normal response to loss. (201.24.c.g.d.m.a.17)

202. The answer is c. Sedating benzodiazepines may help with transitory sleep difficulties and with intense feelings of being overwhelmed. (202.24.c.g.d.t.m.a.17)

203. The answer is e. Acute grief, in general, lasts months beyond the standard expectations or ceremonies that observe grief. (203.24.c.g.d.m.a. 17)

204. The answer is b. Grief is normal. The wound needs to be talked about. (204.24.c.g.t.m.a.17)

205. The answer is e. Pain is difficult to diagnose by use of objective tests. (205.76.c.g.d.m.a.33)

206. The answer is d. The patient's name and address; the name, address, and registration number of the practitioner; the name, strength, and quantity of the drug being dispensed; and the directions for use are all required. (206.76.c.g.p.t.m.a.33)

207. The answer is e. Visceral pain is often described as dull, crampy, and poorly localized, while neuropathic pain may be sharp, shooting, or burning. (207.76.c.g.d.m.a.33)

208. The answer is c. (208.76.c.g.d.m.a.33)

209. The answer is d. (209.76.c.g.d.m.a.33)

210. The answer is b. (210.76.c.g.d.m.a.33)

211. The answer is a. (211.76.c.g.d.m.a.33)

212. The answer is c. Typically a minor injury is responsible for the syndrome. (212.76.c.g.p.t.m.a.33)

213. The answer is d. It can be blocked by serotonin antagonists; for example, ketanserin. (213.76.c.g.p.t.m.a.33)

214. The answer is c. Terfenadine is an antihistamine agent. (214.76.c.g. p.t.m.a.33)

215. The answer is d. 10 milligrams of parenteral methadone is equipotent to 10 mg of parenteral morphine. (215.76.c.g.p.t.m.a.33)

216. The answer is c. This concept was first described by Kahana and Bibring in 1964. (216.45.c.g.d.m.a.32)

217. The answer is a. The other three (not listed) were orderly, superior feeling, and dramatizing. (217.45.c.g.d.m.a.32)

218. The answer is c. Aprosodia may be present, but it is not a listed higher cortical function associated with dementia. (218.7.72.c.g.d.m.a.22)

219. The answer is b. (219.7.72.c.g.d.m.a.22)

220. The answer is a. (220.7.72.c.g.d.m.a.22)

221. The answer is c. (221.7.72.c.g.d.m.a.22)

222. The answer is e. (222.7.72.c.g.d.m.a.22)

223. The answer is d. (223.7.72.c.g.d.m.a.22)

224. The answer is a. By age 85, the prevalence may be as high as 50%. (224.7.63.c.g.d.m.a.22)

225. The answer is true. (225.7.63.c.g.d.f.a.22)

226. The answer is true. (226.7.63.c.g.d.f.a.22)

227. The answer is false. It usually affects the frontal lobes and leads to impairment in executive function and behavior. (227.7.72.c.g.p.d.f.a.22)

228. The answer is false. It is a rapidly progressive disorder. (228.7.c.g. d.f.a.22)

229. The answer is true. (229.7.c.g.d.f.a.22)

230. The answer is false. Tacrine but not donepezil requires monitoring for reversible elevations of liver transaminases. (230.7.c.g.t.f.a.22)

231. The answer is b. (231.72.c.g.d.m.a.23)

232. The answer is a. (232.72.c.g.d.m.a.23)

233. The answer is d. (233.72.c.g.d.m.a.23)

234. The answer is c. (234.72.c.g.d.m.a.23)

235. The answer is e. (235.72.c.g.d.m.a.23)

236. The answer is a. (236.72.c.g.d.m.a.23)

237. The answer is c. (237.72.c.g.d.m.a.23)

238. The answer is e. (238.72.c.g.d.m.a.23)

239. The answer is d. (239.72.c.g.d.m.a.23)

240. The answer is b. (240.72.c.g.d.m.a.23)

241. The answer is b. (241.72.c.g.d.m.a.23)

242. The answer is d. (242.72.c.g.d.m.a.23)

243. The answer is e. (243.72.c.g.d.m.a.23)

244. The answer is a. (244.72.c.g.d.m.a.23)

245. The answer is c. (245.72.c.g.d.m.a.23)

246. The answer is true. (246.72.c.g.d.f.a.23)

247. The answer is true. (247.72.c.g.d.f.a.23)

248. The answer is false. While often drug induced, hallucinations are not stimulated by external stimuli as are illusions. (248.72.c.g.d.f.a.23)

249. The answer is true. (249.61.72.c.g.d.f.a.23)

250. The answer is false. The MMSE is not especially sensitive to frontal lobe functions. (250.61.72.c.g.d.f.a.23)

251. The answer is c. (251.72.c.g.d.m.a.23)

252. The answer is e. (252.72.c.g.d.m.a.23)

253. The answer is a. (253.72.c.g.d.m.a.23)

254. The answer is b. (254.72.c.g.d.m.a.23)

255. The answer is d. (255.72.c.g.d.m.a.23)

256. The answer is d. (256.72.c.g.d.m.a.23)

257. The answer is e. (257.72.c.g.d.m.a.23)

258. The answer is c. (258.72.c.g.d.m.a.23)

259. The answer is b. (259.72.c.g.d.m.a.23)

260. The answer is a. (260.72.c.g.d.m.a.23)

261. The answer is d. (261.12.72.c.g.d.m.a.18)

262. The answer is e. (262.12.72.c.g.d.m.a.18)

263. The answer is b. (263.12.72.c.g.d.m.a.18)

264. The answer is a. (264.12.72.c.g.d.m.a.18)

265. The answer is c. (265.12.72.c.g.d.m.a.18)

266. The answer is a. Visual hallucinations are common in the elderly and in those with sensory/visual problems. (266.72.c.g.d.m.a.18)

267. The answer is c. (267.72.c.g.d.m.a.18)

268. The answer is b. (268.72.c.g.d.m.a.18)

269. The answer is a. (269.72.c.g.d.m.a.18)

270. The answer is a. (270.12.72.c.g.d.m.a.18)

271. The answer is e. (271.12.72.c.g.d.m.a.18)

272. The answer is a. (272.30.c.g.p.t.m.a.18)

273. The answer is b. (273.30.c.g.p.t.m.a.18)

274. The answer is a. (274.63.74.c.g.p.d.m.a.24)

275. The answer is c. (275.74.c.g.d.m.a.24)

276. The answer is c. (276.74.c.g.d.m.a.24)

277. The answer is b. (277.74.c.g.d.m.a.24)

278. The answer is e. By definition, a seizure involving an alteration in consciousness would be at the very least a complex partial seizure. (278. 74.c.g.d.m.a.24)

279. The answer is false. Many, but not all, complex partial seizures originate in the temporal lobe. (279.74.c.g.d.m.a.24)

280. The answer is a. (280.74.c.g.d.m.a.24)

281. The answer is e. Flickering fluorescent lamps, but not incandescent lamps, can induce partial seizures. (281.74.c.g.d.m.a.24)

282. The answer is true. (282.74.c.g.d.f.a.24)

283. The answer is e. Cyclosporine is associated with seizures less than one percent of the time. (283.74.c.g.d.m.a.24)

284. The answer is true. (284.74.c.g.d.f.a.24)

285. The answer is d. Subsequent EEGs with nasopharyngeal leads, or when done in sleep-deprived patients, increases the yield. (285.74.c.g. d.m.a.24)

286. The answer is false. Typically, post-traumatic seizures occur less than one year following an injury. (286.74.c.g.d.f.a.24)

287. The answer is true. The duration is usually more than five minutes. (287.74.c.g.d.f.a.24)

288. The answer is true. (288.74.c.g.d.f.a.24)

289. The answer is false. These characteristics are typical of pseudo-seizures. (289.74.c.g.d.f.a.24)

290. The answer is b. (290.74.c.g.p.t.f.a.24)

291. The answer is b. (291.74.c.g.p.t.m.a.24)

292. The answer is c. (292.74.c.g.p.t.m.a.24)

293. The answer is a. (293.74.c.g.p.t.m.a.24)

294. The answer is e. The yearly incidence of brain injury following concussive syndromes secondary to closed-head injury is greater than the incidence of dementia, epilepsy, multiple sclerosis, Parkinson's disease, schizophrenia, and stroke combined. (294.63.72.c.g.d.m.a.25)

295. The answer is d. (295.72.c.g.d.m.a.25)

296. The answer is a. Other somatic symptoms include fatigue, photo-phobia, hypersensitivity to noise, tinnitus, and decreased tolerance for alcohol. (296.72.c.g.d.m.a.25)

297. The answer is b. Other symptoms include anxiety and personality changes. (297.72.c.g.d.m.a.25)

298. The answer is d. Other symptoms include dyspraxia, a vacuous appearance, and poor motivation. (298.72.c.g.d.m.a.25)

299. The answer is d. Cerebral concussion often causes significant disturbances in social and occupational functioning. In school-age children, the impairment may be manifested by worsening academic performance. (299.72.c.g.d.m.a.25)

300. The answer is d. Brain-injured patients are more susceptible to sedating, hypotensive, and extrapyramidal effects of neuroleptics. (300.72.c.g.d.m.a.25)

301. The answer is true. (301.80.c.g.d.f.a.8)

302. The answer is true. (302.80.c.g.d.f.a.8)

303. The answer is false. Idiosyncratic reactions occur in five percent of cases and include hypotension, nausea, flushing, urticaria, and sometimes anaphylaxis. (303.80.c.g.d.f.a.8)

304. The answer is false. Nonionic contrast material is many times more expensive than ionic contrast material. (304.80.c.g.d.f.a.8)

305. The answer is false. Ionic contrast has a greater risk of side effects. (305.80.c.g.d.f.a.8)

306. The answer is true. (306.80.c.g.d.f.a.8)

307. The answer is true. (307.80.c.g.d.f.a.8)

308. The answer is true. Excellent spatial resolution with CT is less than 1 mm. (308.80.c.g.d.f.a.8)

309. The answer is true. (309.80.c.g.d.f.a.8)

310. The answer is false. (310.80.c.g.d.f.a.8)

311. The answer is false. For these lesions, MRI is more useful. (311.80.c.g.d.f.a.8)

312. The answer is false. Because CT uses ionizing radiation, it is strongly contraindicated in pregnancy. (312.80.c.g.d.f.a.8)

313. The answer is true. (313.80.c.g.d.f.a.8)

314. The answer is false. T-1 images are useful for optimal visualization of normal anatomy, while T-2 weighted images detect areas of pathology. (314.80.c.g.d.f.a.8)

315. The answer is true. (315.80.c.g.d.f.a.8)

316. The answer is true. (316.80.c.g.d.f.a.8)

317. The answer is false. MRI is better than CT for the visualization of the posterior fossa and brainstem. (317.80.c.g.d.f.a.8)

318. The answer is true. (318.80.c.g.d.f.a.8)

319. The answer is true. (319.80.c.g.d.f.a.8)

320. The answer is true. (320.80.c.g.d.f.a.8)

321. The answer is false. Four to 8 mm is the best spatial resolution PET scanning can achieve. (321.80.c.g.d.f.a.8)

322. The answer is false. SPECT's spatial resolution is more than 8 mm, while PET's resolution is 4 to 8 mm. (322.80.c.g.d.f.a.8)

323. The answer is e. Other indications, according to Weinberger's 1984 Criteria for CT Imaging in Psychiatric Diseases, are prolonged catatonia, new-onset affective disorders, or personality changes after the age of 50. (323.80.c.g.d.f.a.8)

324. The answer is true. For amputees, the range is 35–58%, while for stroke it is 25–30%. (324.13.45.63.c.g.d.f.a.50)

325. The answer is c. While it can be helpful, assessment of language skills will usually clarify this. (325.45.c.g.d.m.a.50)

326. The answer is c. Roughly 15% of medical outpatients present to their PCP with a sexual complaint. (326.20.63.c.g.d.m.a.41)

327. The answer is false. While the refractory period in men increases with age, in women there is no refractory period. (327.20.c.g.d.f.a.41)

328. The answer is c. Thioridazine may, however, cause retarded or retrograded ejaculation. (328.20.c.g.p.t.m.a.41)

329. The answer is true. (329.20.c.g.d.f.a.41)

330. The answer is b. Premature ejaculation occurs in 30% of men. (330.20.63.c.g.d.m.a.41)

331. The answer is c. Between 10 and 30% of men of all ages experience erectile dysfunction on a regular basis. (331.20.63.c.g.d.m.a.42)

332. The answer is true. (332.20.63.c.g.d.f.a.42)

333. The answer is true. (333.20.c.g.d.f.a.42)

334. The answer is false. While it does occur roughly every 90 minutes, it occurs during REM sleep, and the frequency decreases with age. (334.20.22.c.g.d.f.a.42)

335. The answer is false. Erectile dysfunction is defined as the inability to retain or maintain a satisfying erection until completion of sexual activity, causing marked distress or interpersonal difficulty. Peyronie's disease involves an erection with a curved shaft secondary to fibrosis. (335.20. c.g.d.f.a.42)

336. The answer is a. Clonidine, like other antihypertensives, can cause erectile dysfunction. (336.20.c.g.d.m.a.42)

337. The answer is false. Failure to conceive after one year of regular sexual intercourse or inability to carry a pregnancy to live birth is the definition of infertility. (337.20.26.c.g.d.f.a.43)

338. The answer is false. Infertility is diagnosed in approximately one of every six couples of child-bearing age. (338.20.26.63.c.g.d.f.a.43)

339. The answer is false. Roughly 10% of women under 25 years of age suffer from infertility. (339.20.c.g.d.f.a.43)

340. The answer is false. Roughly 25% of women between 35 and 40 years of age suffer from infertility. (340.20.26.63.c.g.d.f.a.43)

341. The answer is false. Roughly 50% of infertile patients report occupational and social dysfunction secondary to stress. (341.20.26.63.c.g.d.f.a.43)

342. The answer is true. (342.20.26.63.c.g.d.f.a.43)

343. The answer is false. Between 10 and 50% of women suffer an episode of major depression during the first six months after a spontaneous abortion. (343.20.26.63.c.g.d.f.a.43)

344. The answer is true. (344.20.26.c.g.d.f.a.43)

345. The answer is d. Psychotic episodes are not present, but depressed mood, anger, irritability, and diminished concentration are present. (345.26.c.g.d.m.a.44)

346. The answer is false. Roughly two-thirds of women with premenstrual dysphoric disorder have mood or anxiety disorders. (346.26.63.c.g.d.f.a.44)

347. The answer is false. The diagnosis of menopause requires the cessation of menses for 12 consecutive months. (347.26.c.g.d.f.a.45)

348. The answer is b. (348.26.c.g.d.m.a.45)

349. The answer is true. (349.26.c.g.d.f.a.45)

350. The answer is d. (350.26.c.g.d.m.a.45)

351. The answer is true. (351.26.c.g.d.f.a.45)

352. The answer is true. (352.26.c.g.d.f.a.45)

353. The answer is false. There is no compelling evidence for this notion. (353.26.c.g.d.f.a.45)

354. The answer is false. The prevalence is approximately 10%. (354.13.26.63.c.g.d.f.a.46)

355. The answer is true. (355.13.26.c.g.d.f.a.46)

356. The answer is true. (356.26.65.c.g.d.f.a.46)

357. The answer is true. (357.26.c.g.d.f.a.46)

358. The answer is true. (358.26.30.65.c.g.p.t.f.a.46)

359. The answer is true. (359.26.30.65.c.g.p.t.f.a.46)

360. The answer is true. (360.26.31.65.c.g.p.t.f.a.46)

361. The answer is true. (361.26.31.65.c.g.p.t.f.a.46)

362. The answer is false. There is, however, an increased risk of Ebstein's anomaly. (362.26.32.65.c.g.p.t.f.a.46)

363. The answer is true. (363.26.32.65.c.g.p.t.f.a.46)

364. The answer is false. Approximately 50 to 60% of bipolar women relapse during the acute post-partum period. (364.14.26.c.g.p.t.f.a.46)

365. The answer is true. (365.14.26.c.g.p.t.f.a.46)

366. The answer is false. Roughly five percent of children born to valproic-acid-treated mothers develop neural tube defects. (366.26.33.c.g.p.t.f.a.46)

367. The answer is true. (367.26.32.33.c.g.p.t.f.a.46)

368. The answer is false. The risk of spina bifida after prenatal exposure to carbamazepine is one percent. (368.26.33.65.c.g.p.t.f.a.46)

369. The answer is false. Post-partum blues affects 50 to 75% of post-partum women. (369.26.63.c.g.d.f.a.47)

370. The answer is true. (370.26.63.c.g.d.f.a.47)

371. The answer is false. While post-partum blues do develop within two to three days of delivery, they only last up to two weeks. (371.26.63.c.g.d.f.a.47)

372. The answer is false. Post-partum depression is defined as major depression that develops within four weeks of delivery. (372.26.c.g.d.f.a.47)

373. The answer is true. (373.26.c.g.d.f.a.47)

374. The answer is false. The majority of women with post-partum psychosis are eventually diagnosed as having bipolar disorder or major depression. (374.12.13.26.c.g.d.f.a.47)

375. The answer is false. Women with a history of major depression or bipolar disorder have a 30 to 50% risk for developing a post-partum mood disorder. (375.26.63.c.g.d.f.a.47)

376. The answer is false. There is a 70 to 90% risk of developing recurrent post-partum psychosis in those with a history of post-partum psychosis. (376.26.63.c.g.d.f.a.47)

377. The answer is true. (377.26.63.c.g.d.f.a.47)

378. The answer is false. It is post-partum blues for which reassurance is sufficient; post-partum depression requires more intensive treatment. (378.13.26.c.g.t.f.a.47)

379. The answer is true. (379.26.c.g.t.f.a.47)

380. The answer is true. Lithium levels in breast-fed infants may be nearly 50% of the maternal level, posing a significant risk of lithium toxicity in the infant. (380.26.32.c.g.t.f.a.47)

381. The answer is true. (381.16.c.g.d.f.a.56)

382. The answer is true. (382.16.c.g.d.f.a.56)

383. The answer is true. (383.16.c.g.d.f.a.56)

384. The answer is c. Frequently, a traumatized person will be concerned that he or she is going crazy, but psychosis is not a common outcome. (384.16.c.g.d.m.a.56)

385. The answer is false. Symptoms must last at least two days, persist up to four weeks, and occur within four weeks of the trauma. (385. 16.c.g.d.f.a.56)

386. The answer is true. (386.16.c.g.d.f.a.56)

387. The answer is false. The lifetime risk for developing post-traumatic stress disorder is one to three percent. (387.16.63.c.g.d.f.a.56)

388. The answer is true. (388.16.63.c.g.d.f.a.56)

389. The answer is c. There will be time enough to prepare for chronicity if symptoms persist; do first things first. (389.16.c.g.t.m.a.56)

390. The answer is c. There is no long-term benefit of heavily sedating patients immediately following a trauma. (390.16.c.g.t.m.a.56)

391. The answer is e. In general, hospital caretakers are not mandated reporters. It is the patient's decision to report an assault to the police. However, in assaults involving an elder or a minor, providers are mandated to report the abuse. (391.16.c.g.d.m.a.57)

392. The answer is true. (392.16.c.g.d.f.a.57)

393. The answer is d. Despite the need to make multiple decisions, the clinician should provide information to the patient to help the patient make the appropriate decisions. (393.16.c.g.t.m.a.57)

394. The answer is c. Leave the detective work to the police and avoid detailed descriptions of the assailant. (394.16.c.g.t.m.a.57)

395. The answer is true. In addition, feelings of degradation, anxiety, and depression are experienced. (395.16.c.g.d.f.a.57)

396. The answer is false. One should err on the side of writing too little rather than too much. Inconsistencies in the documentation or indications that the patient's character is questionable may be used against the patient. (396.16.c.g.t.f.a.57)

397. The answer is true. This is because the medical record will probably be entered into evidence in the criminal trial and used against the patient. (397.16.c.g.t.f.a.57)

398. The answer is false. Rape victims may decline to receive treatment, but they should be given enough information to make an informed decision. (398.16.c.g.t.f.a.57)

399. The answer is true. (399.16.c.g.t.f.a.57)

400. The answer is d. Patients with OCD are unlikely to report their symptoms voluntarily. (400.15.63.c.g.d.m.a.19)

401. The answer is true. (401.15.c.g.d.f.a.19)

402. The answer is false. BDD involves an imagined defect in physical appearance that may lead to referral for plastic surgery. (402.15.c.g.d.f.a.19)

403. The answer is true. (403.15.63.c.g.d.f.a.19)

404. The answer is false. Only five to 15% of patients with OCD have OCPD. (404.15.63.c.g.d.f.a.19)

405. The answer is true. (405.15.c.g.d.f.a.19)

406. The answer is d. Among the tricyclic antidepressants (TCAs), clomipramine but not imipramine has been found effective for symptoms of OCD. In general, SSRIs are more effective for OCD symptoms than are the TCAs. (406.15.c.g.p.t.m.a.19)

407. The answer is true. However, even a 50% reduction in symptom severity leads to improved functioning and improved spirits. (407.15.c.g. p.t.f.a.19)

408. The answer is b. (408.14.63.c.g.d.m.a.21)

409. The answer is c. Only 27% of those diagnosed with bipolar disorder are receiving medical treatment. This represents the lowest percentage of any major psychiatric illness. (409.14.63.c.g.p.t.m.a.21)

410. The answer is c. The morbidity, mortality, and disability associated with bipolar mood disorder rank above nearly all other medical disorders. (410.14.63.c.g.p.d.m.a.21)

411. The answer is b. The mean duration of mixed episodes of bipolar disorder is longer, lasting 39 weeks on average. (411.14.c.g.d.m.a.21)

412. The answer is true. (412.14.c.g.d.f.a.21)

413. The answer is c. Other causes of secondary mania include use of steroids or anticholinergic agents, hypoglycemia, electrolyte imbalance, and stroke. (413.9.14.c.g.d.m.a.21)

414. The answer is d. While each of the other choices listed play a role in the management of cyclical mood disorders, lithium or valproic acid are the first-line treatments. (414.14.33.c.g.p.t.m.a.21)

415. The answer is true. (415.14.33.c.g.p.t.f.a.21)

416. The answer is false. At least one year of maintenance treatment is recommended. (416.14.c.g.p.t.f.a.21)

417. The answer is d. Other criteria include distractibility, an increase in goal-directed activity or psychomotor agitation, and an excessive involvement in pleasurable activities. (417.14.c.g.d.m.a.21)

418. The answer is true. (418.14.c.g.p.d.f.a.21)

419. The answer is b. Hepatic dysfunction is not a significant contra-indication because lithium is not metabolized by the liver. (419.14.32.c.g.p.t.m.a.21)

420. The answer is e. (420.32.c.g.p.t.m.a.21)

421. The answer is d. Although headache is not a common symptom of lithium therapy, GI irritation, sedation, and polydipsia do occur. (421.32.c.g.p.t.m.a.21)

422. The answer is e. Liver function tests are generally not recommended because lithium rarely causes hepatitis and is not metabolized by the liver. (422.32.84.c.g.p.t.m.a.21)

423. The answer is d. (423.14.29.c.g.p.t.m.a.21)

424. The answer is c. Elevated liver function tests and dizziness are also noted with valproic acid therapy. (424.33.c.g.p.t.m.a.21)

425. The answer is c. Other side effects of carbamazepine therapy include agranulocytosis, rash, erythema multiforme, Stevens-Johnson syndrome, hyponatremia, edema, systemic lupus erythematosus, arrhythmia, and potential as a teratogen. (425.33.c.g.p.t.m.a.21)

426. The answer is true. (426.21.c.g.d.f.a.20)

427. The answer is c. According to *DSM-IV* criteria for anorexia nervosa, at least three consecutive menstrual cycles are absent. (427.21.c.g.d.m.a.20)

428. The answer is d. Approximately half of patients with anorexia nervosa have bulimic symptoms. (428.21.c.g.d.m.a.20)

429. The answer is c. (429.21.63.c.g.d.m.a.20)

430. The answer is false. Approximately 0.5 percent of adolescent and young adult women suffer from anorexia nervosa, while three percent of adult women have bulimia nervosa. (430.21.63.c.g.d.f.a.20)

431. The answer is false. Up to five percent of patients with anorexia nervosa die from their illness. (431.21.c.g.d.f.a.20)

432. The answer is b. Lanugo is more typically associated with anorexia nervosa. (432.21.c.g.d.m.a.20)

433. The answer is c. Polycystic ovaries are more often associated with temporal lobe epilepsy. (433.21.74.c.g.d.m.a.20)

434. The answer is true. (434.21.c.g.t.f.a.20)

435. The answer is true. Moreover, osteoporosis may not reverse with refeeding. (435.21.c.g.t.f.a.20)

436. The answer is true. (436.21.31.c.g.p.t.f.a.20)

437. The answer is false. While excessive adipose tissue is present, only 120% of ideal body weight is required for the diagnosis of obesity to be made. (437.21.c.g.d.f.a.48)

438. The answer is c. Over $35 billion is spent annually on out-of-pocket weight loss treatments and $75 billion is spent annually on associated health care costs related to obesity. (438.21.c.g.d.m.a.48)

439. The answer is d. In addition, degenerative arthritis, infertility, gall bladder disease, gout, menstrual irregularities, hypothyroidism, polycystic ovarian syndrome, and Cushing's disease are associated with obesity. (439.9.21.c.g.d.m.a.48)

440. The answer is c. (440.30.31.32.c.g.d.t.m.a.48)

441. The answer is false. Testing the stool for phenolphthalein can help identify the patient who has been taking phenolphthalein-containing laxatives (even though these drugs were taken off the U.S. market in 1997). Not all laxatives contain phenolphthalein; some contain magnesium, sorbitol, mineral oil, or motility stimulants. (441.21.c.g.p.d.t.f.a.48)

442. The answer is true. (442.21.63.c.g.p.d.f.a.48)

443. The answer is e. Sibutramine (an anorexiant); dexfenfluramine (Redux), removed from the market due to associated cardiac valvular disease; phentermine (not associated with valvular disease); and phenylpropanolamine (a sympathomimetic) have each led to weight reduction, while cyproheptadine (an antihistamine) is associated with weight gain. (443.21.c.g.p.t.m.a.48)

444. The answer is d. A host of conditions may be AIDS-defining conditions, including HIV encephalopathy. (444.50.c.g.d.m.a.39)

445. The answer is true. (445.50.63.c.g.d.f.a.39)

446. The answer is d. Aspergillosis, coccidioides, cytomegalovirus, herpes simplex, and herpes zoster are also present in HIV-infected patients. (446.9.50.c.g.d.m.a.39)

447. The answer is true. (447.50.c.g.p.d.f.a.39)

448. The answer is b. Depression and irritability may also occur in association with AZT treatment. (448.50.c.g.p.t.m.a.39)

449. The answer is a. Also noted are depersonalization, hyperesthesia, and agitation. (449.50.c.g.p.t.m.a.39)

450. The answer is a. Hypertension is also a side-effect associated with pentamidine treatment. (450.50.c.g.p.t.m.a.39)

451. The answer is true. (451.50.c.g.d.f.a.39)

452. The answer is true. However, up to two-thirds of patients with AIDS-defining illness manifest HIV dementia. (452.7.50.63.c.g.d.f.a.39)

453. The answer is true. (453.34.50.c.g.p.t.f.a.39)

454. The answer is true. (454.50.c.g.p.t..f.a.39)

455. The answer is false. In fact, after AIDS itself, suicide may be the second-leading cause of death among those with HIV and AIDS. (445.38. 50.c.g.d.f.a.39)

456. The answer is true. (456.51.c.g.d.f.a.40)

457. The answer is true. (457.51.c.g.d.f.a.40)

458. The answer is c. Noncompliance may well be a reason to exclude a patient from a transplant list. (458.41.51.c.g.t.m.a.40)

459. The answer is e. (459.51.61.c.g.d.m.a.40)

460. The answer is d. (460.51.c.g.d.m.a.40)

461. The answer is true. (461.31.51.c.g.p.t.f.a.40)

462. The answer is e. Homelessness does not imply severe disturbances or dysfunction. It refers to a person's housing status. (462.52.63.c.g.d. m.a.64)

463. The answer is true. (463.52.c.g.d.f.a.64)

464. The answer is c. Schizophrenia in homeless adults occurs 30 times more often than in matched housed samples. (464.12.52.63.c.g.d.m.a.64)

465. The answer is e. Roughly two-thirds to as many as 90% in some samples of homeless adults abuse alcohol. (465.10.52.63.c.g.d.m.a.64)

466. The answer is true. Chronic lung disease is 15 times more prevalent among the homeless than in those with regular housing. (466.52.63.c. g.d.f.a.64)

467. The answer is b. Roughly 25% of homeless adults report having had psychiatric hospitalizations. (467.52.63.c.g.d.m.a.64)

468. The answer is c. Since memory disorders are not prominent in homeless adults, this factor is least likely to account for noncompliance (468.41.52.c.g.t.m.a.64).

469. The answer is true. (469.52.c.g.d.f.a.64)

470. The answer is true. Complaints by other shelter dwellers may lead to extrusion because of loud snoring. (470.22.52.c.g.d.f.a.64)

471. The answer is false. In fact, homeless persons are generally reassured by explicit promises that their privacy is being protected. (471.39. 52.c.g.t.f.a.64)

472. The answer is e. Renal function is not likely to be more abnormal among the homeless; it falls within the rubric of general medical information. (472.37.52.c.g.d.m.a.64)

473. The answer is true. (473.52.c.g.p.t.f.a.64)

474. The answer is true. (474.25.c.g.t.f.a.65)

475. The answer is true. (475.25.66.c.g.t.f.a.65)

476. The answer is false. Not at all; however, the situation that surrounds a celebrity brings out narcissistic traits both in the staff caring for the celebrity patient and in the family and staff the celebrity brings into the medical environment. (476.25.c.g.d.f.a.65)

477. The answer is c. Business success is not required for the diagnosis of narcissistic personality disorder. (477.25.c.g.d.m.a.65)

478. The answer is true. (478.25.c.g.d.f.a.65)

479. The answer is false. The person who cares for a celebrity should ask the patient explicitly who is to be privy to information and who is not in the loop. (479.25.66.c.g.t.f.a.65)

480. The answer is true. The pseudonym is a tool that should be unique and keyed to only one patient identification number. (480.25.66.c.g.t.f.a. 65)

481. The answer is false. Clinicians often have fantasies; however, these fantasies and wishes should not interfere with clinical behavior. (481.25. 66.c.g.t.f.a.65)

482. The answer is false. Caregivers should not assume that their physician patients have the appropriate knowledge. The best policy is to explain everything in detail preceded by reassurance with "You're probably aware of these factors, but. . . ." (482.25.66.c.g.t.f.a.65)

483. The answer is false. Substance abuse should not be overlooked. Similarly, other health-related factors need to be explored. (483.25.66.c.g. t.f.a.65)

484. The answer is true. (484.47.c.g.t.f.a.59)

485. The answer is false. (485.47.c.g.t.f.a.59)

486. The answer is false. The impact on all the members of the relevant family system acts as the focus for the meeting. (486.47.c.g.t.f.a.59)

487. The answer is true. (487.47.c.g.t.f.a.59)

488. The answer is true. (488.47.c.g.t.f.a.59)

489. The answer is false. The most conservative position is to refer each member of the family unit to individual therapy and the abuser to group treatment. (489.47.53.c.g.t.f.a.59)

490. The answer is false. Even when it has been determined that a psychotic, depressed, anorectic, or chronically mentally ill person's condition has been worsened by family interactions that can be addressed in family therapy, the patient's individual condition must be thoroughly evaluated medically and treated comprehensively. (490.47.c.g.t.f.a.59)

491. The answer is false. One-third to one-half of all marriages involve physical violence. (491.49.63.c.g.d.f.a.58)

492. The answer is false. Nearly one-fifth of homicides occur within the family. (492.49.63.c.g.d.f.a.58)

493. The answer is true. (493.49.63.c.g.d.f.a.58)

494. The answer is false. Abused women have substantially more complaints of these types than do nonabused women. (494.49.63.c.g.d.f.a.58)

495. The answer is true. (495.49.63.c.g.d.f.a.58)

496. The answer is true. (496.10.11.49.63.c.g.d.f.a.58)

497. The answer is true. (497.49.c.g.d.f.a.58)

498. The answer is true. (498.49.c.g.d.f.a.58)

499. The answer is d. (499.49.c.g.d.m.a.58)

500. The answer is true. Usually, abused individuals report information to physicians who question in a tactful, empathic fashion. (500.49.c.g.d.f.a.58)

501. The answer is true. Up to 40% of women who present with trauma have injuries secondary to battery. (501.37.49.c.g.d.f.a.58)

502. The answer is c. Twelve percent. (502.5.63.c.g.d.m.a.30)

503. The answer is false. Those with major difficulties in one area typically have difficulty in other areas as well. (503.5.63.c.g.d.f.a.30)

504. The answer is c. Other areas to be assessed include general health, reaction to stress, quality of attachments, parental competency, family resources, and community resources. (504.4.5.6.c.g.d.m.a.30)

505. The answer is d. Symptoms must be associated with impairment in functioning in at least two settings; that is, home and school. Symptoms must have begun prior to age seven to qualify for the diagnosis. Attentional problems but not hyperactivity can be manifested by impatience, and the prevalence is estimated at five percent in children and two percent in adults. (505.5.63.c.g.d.m.a.31)

506. The answer is false. ADHD persists into adulthood in a substantial number of cases. (506.5.c.g.d.f.31)

507. The answer is true. (507.5.63.c.g.d.f.31)

508. The answer is false. History should be gathered from parents, care-takers, and whenever possible the records of teachers with the permission of the patient or parents. (508.5.c.g.d.f.a.31)

509. The answer is e. Greater than 30% have learning disabilities. (509.5.63.c.g.d.f.a.31)

510. The answer is true. (510.5.34.c.g.p.t.f.a.31)

511. The answer is d. (511.5.34.c.g.p.t.m.a.31)

512. The answer is a. (512.5.34.c.g.p.t.m.a.31)

513. The answer is false. Co-administration of stimulants and tricyclic antidepressants or anticonvulsants has been associated with increases in the serum levels of both medications. (513.5.34.c.g.p.t.f.a.31)

514. The answer is d. Stimulants, MAOIs, TCAs, beta-blockers, and clonidine have all been reported to improve symptoms of ADHD, while calcium channel blockers have not. (514.5.31.34.c.g.p.t.m.a.31)

515. The answer is d. Other conditions associated with cocaine abuse and dependence include depression, panic, hypertension, rupture of the ascending aorta, bronchitis, and abruptio placentae. (515.11.c.g.p.t.m.a. 53)

516. The answer is c. (516.11.c.g.p.t.m.a.53)

517. The answer is true. Cocaine metabolites can be detected two to three days after use, whereas amphetamine metabolites can be detected one to two days after use. (517.11.c.g.p.t.f.a.53)

518. The answer is true. Marijuana metabolites may be detected up to 30 days after use. (518.11.c.g.p.t.f.a.53)

519. The answer is e. While withdrawal is a feature that can be seen after continuous substance use, seizures are not a requirement for the diagnosis. (519.11.c.g.d.m.a.53)

520. The answer is e. Dopamine agonists, such as bromocriptine, amantadine, and mazindol, as well as the tricyclic desipramine, have been found helpful; but beta-blockers, while helpful in the management of acute cocaine intoxication, have not been found beneficial for cocaine craving or withdrawal. (520.11.c.g.p.t.m.a.53)

521. The answer is c. An increased respiratory rate occurs with opiate withdrawal. (521.11.c.g.p.t.m.a.53)

522. The answer is e. Sixty-two percent. It accounts for 12 million people per year in the United States. (522.11.c.g.p.d.m.a.53)

523. The answer is e. Normal-pressure hydrocephalus may be associated with ataxia, incontinence, and confusion, but it is not in general an acute life-threatening illness associated with agitation. (523.6.23.70.c.g.d. m.a.60)

524. The answer is b. The mnemonic WHHHIMP helps to recall the life-threatening causes of agitation or delirium. These include Wernicke's encephalopathy, hypertension, hypoxia, hypoglycemia, intracranial bleeds, meningitis or metabolic derangement, and poisoning. (524.6.23.c.g.d.m.a. 60)

525. The answer is d. (525.23.70.c.g.d.m.a.60)

526. The answer is d. It is wise not to be confrontational or to promise more than you can deliver. Trust is important. (526.23.70.c.g.d.m.a.60)

527. The answer is b. Avoid touching the patient unnecessarily, and during the physical exam tell the patient what you are doing before you do it. (527.23.70.c.g.t.m.a.60)

528. The answer is b. (528.23.70.c.g.d.m.a.60)

529. The answer is true. (529.12.23.70.c.g.d.f.a.60)

530. The answer is false. Safety cannot be over-emphasized. Trust your feelings when you do not feel safe with a patient and take the necessary preventive measures to manage the environment before you continue with the examination. (530.23.70.c.g.d.f.a.60)

531. The answer is true. (531.10.23.70.c.g.d.f.a.60)

532. The answer is b. Also useful in some patients are benzodiazepines, buspirone, and psychostimulants in those with impulsivity associated with ADHD. (532.29.30.31.32.33.c.g.p.d.t.a.60)

533. The answer is b. Other indications include disorders of the neurologic, respiratory, gastrointestinal, renal, endocrine, hematologic, neoplastic, rheumatologic, allergic, dermatologic, and ophthalmologic systems. (533.9.36.37.c.g.p.t.m.a.54)

534. The answer is b. (534.9.36.c.g.p.t.m.a.54)

535. The answer is a. (535.9.36.c.g.p.t.m.a.54)

536. The answer is d. (536.9.36.c.g.p.t.m.a.54)

537. The answer is c. (537.9.36.c.g.p.t.m.a.54)

538. The answer is e. (538.9.36.c.g.p.t.m.a.54)

539. The answer is e. Headache, muscle weakness, aseptic necrosis of the femoral head, sodium retention, hypertension, menstrual irregularities, and manifestations of latent diabetes are also seen with glucocorticoids. (539.9.36.c.g.p.t.m.a.54)

540. The answer is true. Depression and mania each account for roughly one-third of severe psychiatric syndromes, and psychosis and delirium each account for roughly one-sixth of serious psychiatric syndromes. (540.6.9.36.c.g.p.t.f.a.54)

541. The answer is d. Mild euphoria is common as a symptom of steroid treatment, as are insomnia and irritability. (541.9.36.c.g.p.t.m.a.54)

542. The answer is c. Symptoms develop either within hours of initiation of steroid treatment or after several months. (542.36.c.g.p.t.m.a.54)

543. The answer is true. Approximately 60% of glucocorticoid-treated patients with psychiatric symptoms are women. Even when conditions like SLE and rheumatoid arthritis, which occur more commonly in women, are excluded, an estimated 15 to 20% of women who undergo steroid treatment develop neuropsychiatric symptoms, compared with three percent of men. (543.36.c.g.p.t.f.a.54)

544. The answer is false. The vast majority of patients who develop neuropsychiatric difficulties from steroid use have no prior psychiatric illness. (544.36.63.c.g.p.t.f.a.54)

545. The answer is false. (545.36.37.63.c.g.p.t.f.a.54)

546. The answer is false. (546.36.37.63.c.g.p.t.f.a.54)

547. The answer is true. (547.36.37.63.c.g.p.t.f.a.54)

548. The answer is true. (548.36.37.63.c.g.p.t.f.a.54)

549. The answer is d. Twenty percent. (549.36.37.63.c.g.p.t.m.a.54)

550. The answer is e. Slowed mentation, disorientation, and anorexia also occur. (550.36.37.63.c.g.p.t.m.a.54)

551. The answer is e. While many physicians wish to obtain the lowest cost of care for their patients, negotiating about pricing of medications is not standard practice. (551.41.c.g.p.t.m.a.55)

552. The answer is e. At least half of all patients alter the way they take their medications. (552.41.c.g.p.t.m.a.55)

553. The answer is b. (553.31.36.c.g.p.t.m.a.66)

554. The answer is d. (554.31.36.c.g.p.t.m.a.66)

555. The answer is a. (555.31.36.c.g.p.t.m.a.66)

556. The answer is b. (556.31.36.c.g.p.t.m.a.66)

557. The answer is b. (557.31.36.c.g.p.t.m.a.66)

558. The answer is a. (558.31.36.c.g.p.t.m.a.66)

559. The answer is a. (559.31.36.c.g.p.t.m.a.66)

560. The answer is b. (560.31.36.c.g.p.t.m.a.66)

561. The answer is true. (561.31.36.c.g.p.t.f.a.66)

562. The answer is true. (562.31.36.c.g.p.t.f.a.66)

563. The answer is d. Each of the other agents may induce, not treat, a hypotensive crisis in the presence of MAOIs. (563.31.36.c.g.p.t.m.a.66)

564. The answer is a. (564.31.36.c.g.p.t.m.a.66)

565. The answer is a. (565.31.36.c.g.p.t.m.a.66)

566. The answer is a. TCAs with prominent anticholinergic side-effects tend to cause sinus tachycardia. (566.31.36.c.g.p.t.m.a.66)

567. The answer is b. (567.36.c.g.p.t.m.a.66)

568. The answer is b. (568.36.c.g.p.t.m.a.66)

569. The answer is b. Supplementation with pyridoxine (50 to 150 mg at bedtime) may help relieve MAOI-induced pyridoxine deficiency and subsequent paresthesias. (569.36.c.g.p.t.m.a.66)

570. The answer is d. Increased temperature, not decreased temperature, is caused by anti-cholinergic effects. (570.36.c.g.p.t.m.a.66)

571. The answer is b. Each of the other agents can alleviate antidepressant-induced sexual dysfunction. (571.20.31.36.c.g.p.t.m.a.66)

572. The answer is b. Trazodone induces, not treats, priapism. (572.20.31.36.c.g.p.t.m.a.66)

573. The answer is true. (573.31.36.c.g.p.t.f.a.67)

574. The answer is true. However, they may be proarrhythmic in a minority of patients. (574.31.36.c.g.p.t.f.a.67)

575. The answer is false. (575.31.35.36.c.g.p.t.f.a.67)

576. The answer is false. Lithium levels will rise by roughly 25% with use of thiazide diuretics. (576.32.35.36.c.g.p.t.f.a.67)

577. The answer is false. TCAs tend to cause sinus tachycardia. (577.31.36.c.g.p.t.f.a.67)

578. The answer is true. Lithium tends to be associated with sinus node dysfunction and should be avoided in sick sinus syndrome. (578.32.36.c.g.p.t.f.a.67)

579. The answer is false. TCAs should be avoided with second- or third-degree AV block unless a pacemaker is present. (579.31.36.c.g.p.t.f.a.67)

580. The answer is true. These agents should be avoided because of the risk of complete heart block. (580.31.36.c.g.p.t.f.a.67)

581. The answer is true. (581.33.35.36.c.g.p.t.f.a.67)

582. The answer is true. (582.33.35.36.c.g.p.t.f.a.67)

583. The answer is false. (583.30.36.c.g.p.t.f.a.67)

584. The answer is false. Torsade is an alternative name for polymorphic ventricular tachycardia. (584.30.36.c.g.p.t.f.a.67)

585. The answer is false. (585.31.36.c.g.p.t.f.a.67)

586. The answer is false. (586.31.36.c.g.p.t.f.a.67)

587. The answer is true. (587.31.36.c.g.p.t.f.a.67)

588. The answer is true. (588.31.36.c.g.p.t.f.a.67)

589. The answer is false. A QRS complex duration of between 100 to 120 milliseconds is consistent with an intraventricular conduction defect (IVCD); a QRS greater than 120 milliseconds is termed complete bundle branch block. A right bundle branch block has a different pattern than a left bundle branch block. (589.36.c.g.p.t.f.a.67)

590. The answer is true. (590.31.36.c.g.p.t.f.a.67)

591. The answer is true. (591.31.c.g.p.t.f.a.67)

592. The answer is false. Tertiary TCAs include amitriptyline and imipramine; protriptyline is a secondary amine. (592.31.c.g.p.t.f.a.67)

593. The answer is false. Desipramine and nortriptyline are secondary TCAs; trimipramine is a tertiary TCA. (593.31.c.g.p.t.f.a.67)

594. The answer is true. (594.31.36.c.g.p.t.f.a.67)

595. The answer is true. (595.28.30.c.g.p.t.f.a.67)

596. The answer is true. Eight milligrams of perphenazine is the dose equivalent to 5 mg of thiothixene. (596.30.c.g.p.t.f.a.67)

597. The answer is true. (597.30.c.g.p.t.f.a.67)

598. The answer is true. (598.30.c.g.p.t.f.a.67)

599. The answer is false. (599.28.30.c.g.p.t.f.a.67)

600. The answer is false. Up to 25% of patients taking clozapine manifest sinus tachycardia. (600.30.36.c.g.p.t.f.a.67)

601. The answer is true. (601.28.30.c.g.p.t.f.a.67)

602. The answer is true. (602.28.30.c.g.p.t.f.a.67)

603. The answer is true. (603.28.30.c.g.p.t.f.a.67)

604. The answer is true. (604.32.36.c.g.p.t.f.a.67)

605. The answer is true. The half-life for dextroamphetamine is 12 hours, while the half-life for methylphenidate is 4 hours. (605.34.36.c.g.p.t.f.a.67)

606. The answer is true. (606.35.c.g.p.t.f.a.68)

607. The answer is false. Medications with a low therapeutic index have a low margin between a toxic dose and a therapeutic dose. The term has nothing to do with onset of action or rapidity of reaching therapeutic levels. (607.35.c.g.p.t.f.a.68)

608. The answer is true. (608.32.35.c.g.p.t.f.a.68)

609. The answer is true. They are relatively ineffective at doses below or above a specific therapeutic range. (609.35.c.g.p.t.f.a.68)

610. The answer is true. (610.31.35.c.g.p.t.f.a.68)

611. The answer is false. These reactions are unpredictable in a small number of patients and are unexpected from known pharmacokinetic and pharmacologic properties. (611.35.c.g.p.t.f.a.68)

612. The answer is false. Such interactions are pharmacologic, not pharmacokinetic. (6612.35.c.g.p.t.f.a.68)

613. The answer is true. (613.35.c.g.p.t.f.a.68)

614. The answer is false. It accelerates it. (614.30.35.c.g.p.t.f.a.68)

615. The answer is true. (615.35.c.g.p.t.f.a.68)

616. The answer is false. Lithium is minimally protein bound. (616.32.35.c.g.p.t.f.a.68)

617. The answer is false. While ketoconazole, erythromycin, and cimetidine are inhibitors, phenytoin is an inducer. (617.33.35.c.g.p.t.f.a.68)

618. The answer is true. (618.35.c.g.p.t.f.a.68)

619. The answer is true. (619.35.c.g.p.t.f.a.68)

620. The answer is false. They produce a slow decline over days to weeks. (620.35.c.g.p.t.f.a.68)

621. The answer is true. (621.33.35.c.g.p.t.f.a.68)

622. The answer is false. (622.32.35.c.g.p.t.f.a.68)

623. The answer is false. (623.32.35.c.g.p.t.f.a.68)

624. The answer is true. (624.32.35.c.g.p.t.f.a.68)

625. The answer is false. (625.33.35.c.g.p.t.f.a.68)

626. The answer is true. (626.32.35.c.g.p.t.f.a.68)

627. The answer is true. (627.31.33.35.c.g.p.t.f.a.68)

628. The answer is true. (628.31.35.c.g.p.t.f.a.68)

629. The answer is true. (629.30.31.35.c.g.p.t.f.a.68)

630. The answer is false. (630.31.35.c.g.p.t.f.a.68)

631. The answer is true. (631.31.35.c.g.p.t.f.a.68)

632. The answer is true. (632.31.35.c.g.p.t.f.a.68)

633. The answer is true. (633.31.35.c.g.p.t.f.a.68)

634. The answer is true. (634.30.33.35.c.g.p.t.f.a.68)

635. The answer is true. (635.30.35.c.g.p.t.f.a.68)

636. The answer is c. Jumping to conclusions about the nature of the problem is not a goal of time-limited interviewing. (636.2.c.g.d.m.a.3)

637. The answer is d. Clarify the patient's main concerns and major requests of the physician. Do not make assumptions. (637.2.c.g.d.m.a.3)

638. The answer is a. It is easy to step into closed-ended questions, but this often leads to premature closure regarding data that might otherwise impact on the social or psychological aspects of the situation. (638.2.c. g.d.m.a.3)

639. The answer is a. (639.2.c.g.d.m.a.3)

640. The answer is c. CBT is structured and portions of sessions are devoted to specific interventions or homework assignments. (640.56.57.c. g.t.m.a.9)

641. The answer is true. (641.56.57.c.g.t.f.a.9)

642. The answer is e. Self-monitoring is a significant part of CBT. (642.56.57.c.g.t.m.a.9)

643. The answer is d. It rarely helps to terminate a session before anxiety develops. Instead, anxiety and control of anxiety are required for behavioral change. (643.56.57.c.g.t.m.a.9)

644. The answer is true. (644.56.57.c.g.t.f.a.10)

645. The answer is true. (645.56.57.c.g.t.f.a.10)

646. The answer is false. Repeated exposure without performing compulsions leads to a decrease in anxiety over time. (646.56.57.c.g.t.f.a.10)

647. The answer is false. CBT is at least as effective as medication for OCD, but for patients with severe symptoms a combination of CBT and medication is recommended. (647.56.57.c.g.t.f.a.10)

648. The answer is true. However, benzodiazepine therapy may be preferred to help an individual cope with a feared event that is rarely encountered. (648.56.57.c.g.t.f.a.10)

649. The answer is false. Systematic desensitization refers to a procedure of relaxation training accompanied by gradual exposure (frequently imagined) to a feared stimulus. (649.56.57.c.g.t.f.a.10)

650. The answer is a. (650.41.56.57.c.g.t.m.a.71)

651. The answer is d. (651.41.56.57.c.g.t.m.a.71)

652. The answer is b. (652.41.56.57.c.g.t.m.a.71)

653. The answer is e. (653.41.56.57.c.g.t.m.a.71)

654. The answer is c. (654.41.56.57.c.g.t.m.a.71)

655. The answer is false. (655.56.57.c.g.t.f.a.71)

656. The answer is true. (656.41.c.g.t.f.a.71)

657. The answer is true. (657.56.57.c.g.t.f.a.71)

658. The answer is true. (658.56.57.c.g.t.f.a.71)

659. The answer is true. (659.41.c.g.t.f.a.74)

660. The answer is d. Twenty-five percent of the time medication is stopped after several days. (660.41.c.g.t.m.a.74)

661. The answer is b. Patients do not comply with long-term treatment 50% of the time. (661.41.c.g.t.m.a.74)

662. The answer is true. (662.41.c.g.t.f.a.74)

663. The answer is d. Greater clarity is needed. Patients need to know when and why they need to return for an appointment. (663.41.c.g. t.m.a.74)

664. The answer is true. (664.41.c.g.t.f.a.72)

665. The answer is false. Approximately one-half of American smokers have quit. The vast majority have stopped on their own. (665.41.c.g.t.f.a.72)

666. The answer is false. Approximately two-thirds of those who have quit smoking resume smoking within 3 months. (666.41.c.g.t.f.a.72)

667. The answer is c. Acupuncture appears to be ineffective as a treatment for smoking cessation. (667.41.c.g.t.f.a.72)

668. The answer is b. Decreased sleep as well as decreased concentration, anger, and anxiety accompany nicotine withdrawal. (668.41.c.g.p.t.f.a.72)

669. The answer is true. (669.41.c.g.p.t.f.a.72)

670. The answer is true. (670.41.c.g.p.t.f.a.72)

671. The answer is d. Insomnia rather than excessive daytime sleepiness is a symptom of nicotine toxicity. (671.41.c.g.p.t.m.a.72)

672. The answer is false. The proper formula for calculation of BMI is weight in pounds times 700 divided by height in inches squared. BMIs of 18.9 to 24.9 are ideal. (672.21.c.g.d.f.a.73)

673. The answer is true. (673.21.c.g.t.f.a.73)

674. The answer is false. It is as beneficial. (674.21.c.g.t.f.a.73)

675. The answer is true. (675.25.c.g.d.f.a.12)

676. The answer is true. (676.25.c.g.d.f.a.12)

677. The answer is true. (677.25.c.g.d.f.a.12)

678. The answer is true. (678.25.66.c.g.d.f.a.12)

679. The answer is b. (679.25.c.g.d.m.a.12)

680. The answer is a. (680.25.c.g.d.m.a.12)

681. The answer is true. In the hospital or doctor's office, the dependent individual attempts to wrest from the medical relationship that which he or she did not get from the mother-child relationship. (681.25.c.g.d.f.a.12)

682. The answer is false. The physician should practice repetitive appeals to the patient's sense of entitlement and say something to the effect of, "You deserve the best medical care we can give; that's why we are recommending A, B, and C." (682.25.c.g.t.f.a.12)

683. The answer is false. A balance between healthy denial and pathological denial is needed. Caregivers should confront the most dangerous aspects of denial without feeling responsible for it. (683.25.c.g.t.f.a.12)

684. The answer is true. (684.25.c.g.d.f.a.13)

685. The answer is true. (685.25.c.g.d.f.a.13)

686. The answer is false. It is far more likely that an approach that says, "You don't know me; why should you trust me?" will generate more respect and cooperation. (686.25.c.g.t.f.a.13)

687. The answer is false. If the physician feels depressed and de-skilled, it is far more likely that he or she is dealing with a manipulative help-rejecter. (687.25.c.g.t.f.a.13)

688. The answer is true. (688.25.c.g.t.f.a.13)

689. The answer is e. Although anxiety disorders are more prevalent than the other conditions listed, they tend not to be as disturbing or as disruptive. (689.60.c.g.t.m.a.4)

690. The answer is true. (690.60.c.g.t.f.a.4)

691. The answer is false. Patients are likely to find referral to a known colleague as reassuring, and it allows for better linkage of communication. (691.60.66.c.g.t.f.a.4)

692. The answer is false. Mental health providers are put at a disadvantage if the referred patient has not explicitly made the appointment for reasons with which he or she agrees. (692.60.c.g.t.f.a.4)

693. The answer is false. Certain situations (e.g., impending or imminent suicide or homicide) require psychiatric assessment, treatment, and the provision of a safe environment. (693.60.c.g.t.f.a.4)

694. The answer is true. The prevalence of depression in primary care settings is six to 17%, while it is six percent for hypertension. (694.13.60.c.g.d.f.a.1)

695. The answer is false. 11 to 25% is the prevalence of anxiety disorders in the general population. However, in a given year, only one-third of those with anxiety disorders obtain treatment, and only 15% obtain mental health services. (695.15.60.c.g.d.f.a.1)

696. The answer is true. (696.13.60.c.g.d.f.a.1)

697. The answer is c. Often patients believe that psychiatric care is too expensive and that psychotropics are mind-altering or addictive. (697.60.c.g.d.t.m.a.1)

698. The answer is c. Stampedes like this would be highly unlikely; treatment and referral should be done on a case-by-case basis. (698.60.c.g.t.m.a.1)

699. The answer is true. (699.60.c.g.t.f.a.1)

700. The answer is c. In general, continuity works better than does rotating personnel. (700.60.c.g.t.fm.a.1)

701. The answer is true. (701.58.c.g.d.f.a.2)

702. The answer is false. Behavior therapy is based on reducing symptoms by learning relaxation techniques, changing factors that reinforce symptoms, and giving the patient graduated exposure to distressing stimuli. Behavior therapists are directive and encourage homework experimentation. (702.56.57.c.g.t.f.a.2)

703. The answer is true. (703.56.c.g.t.f.a.2)

704. The answer is false. Interpersonal therapy addresses relationships in the here and now that may contribute to depression. (704.56.c.g.t.a.2)

705. The answer is false. Often care of selected medical populations (e.g., patients with coronary artery disease or cancer) is conducted in such a fashion. (705.48.c.g.t.f.a.2)

706. The answer is false. Signing of a form titled "Informed Consent" does not constitute informed consent. (706.39.c.g.t.f.a.5)

707. The answer is true. (707.39.c.g.t.f.a.5)

708. The answer is b. A health care proxy can provide informed consent. (708.39.c.g.t.m.a.5)

709. The answer is true. (709.39.c.g.t.f.a.5)

710. The answer is true. (710.39.c.g.t.f.a.5)

711. The answer is true. (711.39.c.g.t.f.a.5)

712. The answer is false. Informed consent is both an ethical and a legal obligation. (712.39.c.g.t.f.a.5)

713. The answer is true. (713.39.c.g.d.f.a.5)

714. The answer is false. Certain conditions interfere with a patient's judgment (e.g., psychosis, pain, depression), allowing for a substituted judgment to be invoked. (714.39.c.g.t.f.a.5)

715. The answer is true. (715.39.c.g.d.f.a.5)

716. The answer is false. Only a judge can declare a patient incompetent. (716.39.c.g.d.t.f.a.5)

717. The answer is true. (717.39.c.g.t.f.a.5)

718. The answer is false. Clinical assessment has no effect on a patient's legal status, although it can serve as an indication of the likely outcome of legal proceedings. (718.39.c.g.d.f.a.5)

719. The answer is true. (719.39.c.g.d.f.a.5)

720. The answer is true. (720.39.c.g.d.f.a.5)

721. The answer is true. (721.39.c.g.d.f.a.5)

722. The answer is true. (722.39.c.g.d.f.a.5)

723. The answer is e. While the presence of minor children may allow the treating physicians with court approval to follow a different course of action than desired by the patient, this is not something that prevents a capacity decision from being made. (723.39.c.g.d.f.a.5)

724. The answer is true. (724.39.c.g.d.f.a.5)

725. The answer is true. (725.39.c.g.d.f.a.5)

726. The answer is false. The professional standard is the amount of information a reasonable professional would provide in similar circumstances, while the materiality standard is what the average patient would need in order to come to a decision under the same circumstances. (726.39.c.g.d.f.a.5)

727. The answer is b. The cost, while important, is not a requirement of information provision. (727.39.c.g.t.f.a.5)

728. The answer is false. Informed consent is required. The question is when informed consent should be written in the medical record. If written consent is not required, a verbal discussion with the patient or decision-making person is sufficient. (728.39.c.g.t.f.a.5)

729. The answer is true. (729.39.c.g.t.f.a.5)

730. The answer is true. However, this privilege should be invoked rarely. (730.39.c.g.t.f.a.5)

731. The answer is true. (731.39.c.g.t.f.a.5)

732. The answer is true. It is not necessary, but it is useful to document such questions. (732.39.c.g.t.f.a.5)

733. The answer is false. Involuntary commitment in most states does not mean that the patient can be forced to accept treatment. (733.39.c.g.t.f.a.61)

734. The answer is true. (734.39.c.g.d.f.a.61)

735. The answer is true. (735.39.c.g.d.f.a.61)

736. The answer is false. The need for treatment in the absence of dangerousness is not sufficient. (736.39.c.g.t.f.a.61)

737. The answer is true. (737.39.c.g.d.f.a.61)

738. The answer is false. The presumption of competency persists until a court has declared a person to be incompetent. (738.39.c.g.d.f.a.61)

739. The answer is true. Individuals who are determined to kill themselves may avoid telling those who could put them into a hospital. Further information and protection are required. (739.39.c.g.d.f.a.61)

740. The answer is true. (740.39.c.g.t.f.a.61)

741. The answer is true. (741.39.c.g.t.f.a.61)

742. The answer is true. (742.3.c.g.d.f.6)

743. The answer is e. Effective treatment of the patient is the goal. (743.61.c.g.d.m.a.7)

744. The answer is c. (744.61.c.g.d.m.a.7)

745. The answer is d. By definition, a screen cannot be comprehensive, it can only be a screen. (745.61.c.g.d.m.a.7)

746. The answer is c. (746.61.c.g.d.m.a.7)

747. The answer is a. (747.61.c.g.d.m.a.7)

748. The answer is d. (748.61.c.g.d.m.a.7)

749. The answer is b. (749.61.c.g.d.m.a.7)

750. The answer is e. (750.61.c.g.d.m.a.7)

751. The answer is b. (751.61.c.g.d.m.a.7)

752. The answer is d. (752.61.c.g.d.m.a.7)

753. The answer is c. (753.61.c.g.d.m.a.7)

754. The answer is e. (754.61.c.g.d.m.a.7)

755. The answer is a. (755.61.c.g.d.m.a.7)

756. The answer is c. The frontal lobes, not the limbic system, are thought to regulate executive functions. (756.27.c.g.d.m.f.75)

757. The answer is true. (757.27.71.c.g.d.f.f.75)

758. The answer is true. However, in coma, the arm will drop on the face. (758.71.c.g.d.f.f.75)

759. The answer is false. A boundary crossing—a minor but potentially important blurring of the boundaries—is less severe than the boundary violation, in which the boundaries are clearly transgressed. (759.66.c.g.d.f.a.76)

760. The answer is true. For example, in a rural area, it may be appropriate for the family doctor to spend time with patients at a social gathering, while the same social gathering in an urban practice may be considered a boundary crossing. (760.66.c.g.d.f.a.76)

761. The answer is true. (761.66.c.g.d.f.a.76)

762. The answer is true. (762.66.c.g.d.f.a.76)

763. The answer is false. The APA declared it unethical for a psychiatrist to have a sexual relationship with either a former or current patient. (763.66.c.g.t.f.a.76)

764. The answer is true. (764.66.c.g.d.f.a.76)

765. The answer is true. (765.66.c.g.t.f.a.76)

766. The answer is false. It is a boundary crossing, and it may invite further boundary violations or cause the patient great distress. (766.66.c.g.t.f.a.76)

767. The answer is true. (767.66.c.g.t.f.a.76)

768. The answer is true. (768.66.c.g.t.f.a.76)

769. The answer is false. It is always the physician's responsibility to maintain appropriate boundaries. (769.66.c.g.t.f.a.76)

770. The answer is true. (770.66.c.g.t.f.a.76)

771. The answer is false. The physician should let the patient know that such events are not a normal part of treatment and should not have occurred. Consultation with a colleague or someone who has experience in this area is appropriate. (771.66.c.g.t.f.a.76)

772. The answer is b. Increasing availability and acceptance of somatic symptoms leads to a reduced frequency of health care use two years following employment of such a plan. (772.67.c.g.t.m.a.77)

773. The answer is true. (773.67.c.g.t.f.a.77)

774. The answer is a. Technology to increase access to knowledge should decrease and not increase stress. (774.68.c.g.d.m.a.78)

775. The answer is c. Stress is high, but it does not lead to a of 20% leave of absence rate. (775.68.c.g.d.m.a.78)

776. The answer is b. While time consuming, developing roots and relationships potentially leads to enhanced life experiences and satisfaction. (776.68.c.g.d.m.a.78)

777. The answer is c. Far more likely than a lack of dream recall are gastrointestinal distress, verbal incontinence, irregular sleep and eating habits, disrupted family relationships, and difficulties with memory and concentration. (777.68.c.g.d.m.a.78)

778. The answer is d. Minimization tends to allow the problem to fester, not to resolve it. (778.68.c.g.t.m.a.78)

779. The answer is c. While not insignificant, tics are less serious than the other conditions listed. (779.68.c.g.t.m.a.78)

780. The answer is d. The neurologic substrate for confusion is inattention. Attention refers to the ability of the person to sort out and organize a variety of sensory inputs and potential motor outputs so that thoughts or actions can proceed in a logical fashion. (780.2.6.72.c.g.d.m.d.1)

781. The answer is c. In stupor, there is little or no response to verbal comments, no verbal responses are elicited, and motor responses are defensive or reflexive. (781.2.6.72.c.g.d.m.d.1)

782. The answer is b. (782.71.c.g.d.m.d.1)

783. The answer is d. (783.71.c.g.d.m.d.1)

784. The answer is a. (784.71.c.g.d.m.d.1)

785. The answer is e. (785.71.c.g.d.m.d.1)

786. The answer is c. (786.71.c.g.d.m.d.1)

787. The answer is b. It is respiratory alkalosis (e.g., from hepatic encephalopathy or salicylate poisoning) that causes coma with hyperventilation. (787.44.71.72.c.g.d.m.d.1)

788. The answer is true. Just the reverse is true in pontine lesions, in which the eyes deviate toward the hemiparesis and away from the lesion. (788.71.72.77.c.g.d.f.d.1)

789. The answer is true. By contrast, midposition (approximately 3 to 5 mm) nonreactive pupils are evidence of midbrain damage. (789.71.72.77c.g.d.f.d.1)

790. The answer is d. (790.71.72.c.g.d.m.d.1)

791. The answer is true. (791.71.72.c.g.d.f.d.1)

792. The answer is false. The movement of the eyes described is the slow phase of nystagmus. The fast phase is the corrective movement generated from the frontal lobe contralateral to the direction of the slow phase. (792.71.72.c.g.d.f.d.1)

793. The answer is true. In conscious patients, the vestibulo-ocular reflex is, or can be, suppressed. (793.71.72.c.g.d.f.d.1)

794. The answer is true. (794.71.72.c.g.d.f.d.1)

795. The answer is c. Approximately 25% of migraine sufferers recall childhood vomiting or motion sickness. In addition, 60 to 75% of migraineurs are women. (795.75.c.g.d.m.d.2)

796. The answer is e. Typically, cluster headaches occur without a pro-drome. (796.75.c.g.d.m.d.2)

797. The answer is e. Men are affected by cluster headaches five times more often than are women. (797.63.75.c.g.d.m.d.2)

798. The answer is d. (798.44.71.c.g.d.m.d.2)

799. The answer is e. (799.44.71.c.g.d.m.d.2)

800. The answer is b. (800.44.71.c.g.d.m.d.2)

801. The answer is a. (801.44.71.c.g.d.m.d.2)

802. The answer is c. Stiff neck may also be a sign of meningitis or cer-vical arthritis. (802.44.71.c.g.d.m.d.2)

803. The answer is true. Sumatriptan is also effective in relief of the nau-sea associated with migraine. (803.75.c.g.p.t.f.d.2)

804. The answer is d. Calcium channel blockers, anticonvulsants, and ergotamines are of only minimal benefit in migraine prevention. (804.75. c.g.p.t.m.d.2)

805. The answer is d. Ergotamines are also contraindicated in peripheral vascular disease. (805.75.c.g.p.t.m.d.2)

806. The answer is true. (806.82.c.g.d.f.d.3)

807. The answer is false. Mild mental retardation is associated with IQs between 50 and 70, while severe mental retardation is associated with IQs less than 50. (807.8.82.c.g.d.f.d.3)

808. The answer is true. (808.7.71.72.c.g.d.f.d.3)

809. The answer is b. If the ALT rises to more than five times the upper limit of normal, tacrine should be discontinued. (809.7.c.g.p.t..m.d.3)

810. The answer is true. (810.7.72.c.g.d.f.d.3)

811. The answer is false. Dysequilibrium is defined as a sense of imbalance, unsteadiness, or drunkenness without vertigo. (811.71.72.c.g.d.f.d.4)

812. The answer is d. Peripheral, central, and cardiac causes of dizziness are known, as is orthostatic hypotension. (812.71.72.c.g.d.m.d.4)

813. The answer is d. Ménière's disease is a peripheral cause of dizziness. (813.71.72.c.g.d.m.d.4)

814. The answer is d. Hyperventilation may cause ill-defined giddiness and symptoms other than vertigo, syncope, or dysequilibrium. (814.71.72. c.g.d.m.d.4)

815. The answer is d. (815.71.72.c.g.p.t.m.d.4)

816. The answer is e. (816.71.72.c.g.p.t.m.d.4)

817. The answer is true. (817.9.13.71.76.c.g.d.f.d.5)

818. The answer is true. (818.74.c.g.d.f.d.6)

819. The answer is d. Complex partial seizures are a type of partial seizure, not generalized seizure. (819.74.c.g.d.m.d.6)

820. The answer is true. The EEG is often normal even in patients with known seizure disorders. An abnormal EEG in the absence of seizures does not automatically indicate treatment for seizures. (820.74.84.c.g.d.f.d.6)

821. The answer is c. The patient is rarely aware of these attacks. (821. 74.c.g.d.m.d.6)

822. The answer is d. Carbamazepine decreases phenytoin levels, as does chronic alcohol abuse or use of reserpine. (822.29.33.34.74.c.g.p.t.m.d.6)

823. The answer is d. A body temperature less than 90° Fahrenheit may create an isoelectric EEG, and established cerebral lesion and adequate observation time and apnea are also criteria for brain death. (823.44. 71.72.73.c.g.d.m.d.7)

824. The answer is false. The Jarisch-Herxheimer reaction is a febrile response believed to be caused by the release of large amounts of treponemal products into the circulation after the first 24 hours of therapy. (824.71.c.g.d.f.d.8)

825. The answer is d. This reaction is characterized by decreased blood pressure, fever, tachycardia, and increased white blood cell count that usually begins within 2 hours after the first doses of antibiotics, peaks at 7 hours, and lasts as long as 24 hours. During the reaction, the rash of secondary syphilis, if present, may worsen. (825.71.c.g.d.m.8)

826. The answer is true. (826.74.c.g.d.f.d.9)

827. The answer is true. (827.71.7.2.75.c.g.d.f.d.10)

828. The answer is a. Approximately 5000 new cases of malignant gliomas are discovered each year in the United States. The peak age for malignant gliomas is 45 to 50 years, with men being afflicted more often than women. (828.44.71.7.2.c.g.d.m.d.11)

829. The answer is e. An increase in cerebral edema may also occur. (829.44.71.72.c.g.s.m.d.11)

830. The answer is e. The reverse order is true. (830.71.72.80.c.g.d.m. d.12)

831. The answer is e. Steroids have not been shown to be dramatically effective in most head-injured patients. In addition, side-effects secondary to steroids are common. (831.71.72.c.g.t.m.d.12)

832. The answer is c. Oligoclonal bands are present in 85 to 95% of patients with MS. (832.71.72.84.c.g.d.m.d.13)

833. The answer is c. MRI is better than CT for the detection of CNS demyelination. (833.71.72.73.80.84.c.g.d.m.d.13)

834. The answer is c. Vitamin B_{12} deficiency is not correlated with MS, but the symptoms of B_{12} deficiency are often similar to those of MS. (834.71.72.c.g.d.m.d.13)

835. The answer is d. (835.71.c.g.d.m.d.14)

836. The answer is c. Seizures, coma, and death as well as constipation and anemia are all present in lead toxicity. (836.71.c.g.d.m.d.14)

837. The answer is c. Subacute demyelination of white matter occurs one to three weeks after carbon monoxide exposure. (837.71.c.g.d.m.d.14)

838. The answer is d. Physostigmine is a cholinergic agent, not an anti-cholinergic agent. (838.44.c.g.p.t.m.d.14)

839. The answer is e. Immediate folate administration may cause neurologic deficits, and therefore folate should be withheld until cobalamin stores are repleted over one to two weeks of daily cobalamin injection. (839.71.72.c.g.p.d.t.m.d.14)

840. The answer is e. Benzodiazepines, but not tricyclic antidepressants, can be effective for spasticity. (840.29.31.78.c.g.p.t.m.d.15)

841. The answer is false. Bromocriptine is a dopamine D_2 receptor agonist. (841.28.c.g.p.t.f.d.15)

842. The answer is d. The genetic defect of Huntington's disease is a repeated replication sequence on chromosome 4. (842.78.c.g.d.m.d.15)

843. The answer is a. Wilson's disease is an autosomal recessive disorder. (843.78.c.g.d.m.d.15)

844. The answer is e. (844.82.c.g.d.m)

845. The answer is d. (845.82.c.g.d.m)

846. The answer is c. The Wisconsin Card Sorting Test helps clarify the patient's ability to maintain or shift set. (846.72.82.c.g.d.m)

847. The answer is e. (847.2.72.c.g.d.m)

848. The answer is c. (848.82.c.g.d.m)

849. The answer is e. The MMPI has a true-false format. (849.81.c.g.d.m)

850. The answer is e. Executive function is a frontal, not parietal, lobe function. (850.72.81.c.g.d.m)

851. The answer is c. (851.7.13.74.82.c.g.d.m)

852. The answer is a. However, Mesmer, Freud, and Charcot all used hypnosis. Franklin was a critic of Mesmer's claims. (852.69.c.g.d.m)

853. The answer is a. (853.69.c.g.d.m)

854. The answer is b. Hypnosis is least likely to be successful in demented patients because those with dementia have difficulty with concentration and the use of visual imagery. (854.69.c.g.d.m)

855. The answer is b. (855.69.c.g.t.m)

856. The answer is b. Hypnosis is relatively contraindicated in the paranoid patient, not because it will not work, but because the paranoid patient may blame the practitioner for control of his or her mind. (856.69.c.g.t.m)

857. The answer is c. (857.13.37.44.45.63.c.g.d.m)

858. The answer is c. (858.37.38.44.45.63.c.g.d.m)

859. The answer is e. Morphine is an emetic, not an anti-emetic treatment. (859.36.44.c.g.p.d.m)

860. The answer is e. It is far more likely that hypercalcemia, and not hypocalcemia, with lethargy will be confused with depression in a cancer patient. (860.13.44.45.c.g.d.m)

861. The answer is c. (861.24.37.44.45.63.c.g.d.m)

862. The answer is d. Stimulants are not a treatment for anxiety. If used, they may increase anxiety in this population. (862.15.29.30.34.45.63.c.g. p.t.m)

863. The answer is c. (863.37.44.c.g.d.m)

864. The answer is d. (864.24.44.c.g.d.m)

865. The answer is b. (865.44.c.g.d.m)

866. The answer is b. (866.39.40.44.c.g.d.m)

867. The answer is a. (867.44.c.g.p.d.m)

868. The answer is d. Rash is associated with either primary or secondary syphilitic infection. (868.37.44.71.c.g.d.m)

869. The answer is b. (869.37.44.71.c.g.d.m)

870. The answer is true. (870.37.44.84.c.g.d.f)

871. The answer is true. (871.37.44.84.c.g.d.f)

872. The answer is true. (872.37.44.84.c.g.d.f)

873. The answer is true. (873.37.44.84.c.g.d.f)

874. The answer is c. (874.37.44.71.c.g.d.m)

875. The answer is d. (875.25.c.g.d.m)

876. The answer is c. (876.25.c.g.d.m)

877. The answer is g. (877.25.c.g.d.m)

878. The answer is b. (878.25.c.g.d.m)

879. The answer is f. (879.25.c.g.d.m)

880. The answer is a. (880.25.c.g.d.m)

881. The answer is e. (881.25.c.g.d.m)

882. The answer is d. (882.25.c.g.d.m)

883. The answer is e. (883.25.63.c.g.d.m)

884. The answer is d. (884.25.c.g.d.m)

885. The answer is d. Differential diagnosis, along with a summary of impressions and a formulation of dynamics, are crucial to the psychiatric consultation note, but the use of psychiatric terminology may distance the consultant from the consultee. (885.44.c.g.d.m)

886. The answer is d. The interview of the patient is and should be carried out by the psychiatric consultant. One should not rely solely on the history and documentation performed by others. (886.44.c.g.d.m)

887. The answer is e. Speech rate, production, and latency are all important aspects of assessment of language, while interpretation of proverbs is not part of the language assessment. (887.37.44.71.72.c.g.d.m)

888. The answer is e. While billing codes based on the consultation note are submitted, the psychiatric consultation note is not routinely submitted for reimbursement. (888.44.c.g.t.m)

889. The answer is e. Assessment of competency usually involves assessment of the mental status, but the mental status examination itself does not test for capacity or competency. (889.2.39.40.c.g.d.m)

890. The answer is e. Specific recommendations are usually preferred over general recommendations. (890.44.c.g.t.m)

891. The answer is c. Psychiatric consultants should give medical advice and leave the provision of legal advice to attorneys. (891.39.40.44.c.g.t.m)

892. The answer is c. Psychiatric consultants usually treat the patient and do not commonly treat family members. (892.37.44.c.g.t.m)

893. The answer is d. Discharge is usually left to the consultee. (893.37.44.c.g.t.m)

894. The answer is e. While cognitive assessments and behavioral management of dementia are common, usually these are not emergency consultations. (894.6.7.28.37.39.40.44.c.g.t.m.e)

895. The answer is e. While the liaison psychiatrist may get involved in clinical research, it is not his or her primary function. (895.37.40.c.g.t.m.e)

896. The answer is c. (896.44.c.g.d.m)

897. The answer is d. Competency is not part of the mental status examination but is an important part of the psychiatric consultant's job. (897.2.39.40.44.c.g.d.m)

898. The answer is e. (898.2.72.c.g.d.m)

899. The answer is c. Practice medicine and leave legal strategizing to attorneys. (899.44.c.g.t.m)

900. The answer is c. Family members are generally referred to others rather than having a psychiatric consultant see both the patient and the family member. (900.39.40.44.c.g.t.m)

901. The answer is d. While paralytic agents rarely treat delirium per se, they do allow management of the exceedingly agitated patient along with adequate sedation. By contrast, addition of anticholinergic agents often increases delirium, rather than treating it. (901.6.29.30.c.g.p.t.m)

902. The answer is d. Agitation, memory deficits, inattention, and dysgraphia are each characteristic of delirium, whereas aphasia is rarely seen in delirium. (902.6.71.72.c.g.d.m)

903. The answer is a. Excessive motor activity is the hallmark of agitation. However, many patients who are agitated are also delirious and may manifest hallucinations and disorientation along with attentional and memory deficits. (903.6.71.72.c.g.d.m)

904. The answer is c. Among certain units within the general hospital, especially coronary care units, medical intensive care units, and burn units, and post–cardiac surgery patients, this rate will increase toward 25%. (904.6.44.63.c.g.d.m)

905. The answer is a. Burn patients have the highest reported prevalence and incidence of delirium. Others in intensive care units follow closely behind. (905.6.44.c.g.d.m)

906. The answer is e. (906.6.44.c.g.p.t.m)

907. The answer is b. (907.6.c.g.d.m)

908. The answer is a. (908.6.73.84c.g.d.m)

909. The answer is b. While still uncommon even with high-dose intravenous neuroleptics, Torsade is a potentially lethal cardiac arrhythmia. (909.30.36.44.c.g.p.t.m)

910. The answer is c. While each of these conditions is potentially lethal, hyperkalemia is not a cause for delirium in and of itself, whereas each of the other conditions commonly cause delirium. (910.6.35.44.c.g.t.m)

911. The answer is false. Triphasic delta waves are typically seen in hepatic encephalopathy, whereas low-voltage beta waves are seen in cases of delirium tremens. (911.6.44.73.c.g.d.f)

912. The answer is c. Fluctuations in cognition and behavior are typical of delirium, whereas irreversible organic mental changes and impaired long-term memory are common with dementia, and neologisms and systematic delusions are commonly associated with schizophrenia and other thought disorders. (912.6.44.c.g.d.m)

913. The answer is d. (913.14.44.c.g.p.d.m)

914. The answer is e. SSRIs are infrequently associated with the onset of delirium. (914.31.44.c.g.p.t.m)

915. The answer is e. Myoclonus is exceedingly common in cases of normeperidine toxicity. (915.6.35.36.37.44.c.g.d.m)

916. The answer is a. Intramuscular administration of neuroleptics is associated with the highest rate of extrapyramidal side-effects. (916.30.78. c.g.p.t.m)

917. The answer is e. It is mydriasis, not miosis, that is present in anti-cholinergic delirium. (917.6.35.36.c.g.p.d.m)

918. The answer is b. (918.7.63.c.g.d.m)

919. The answer is c. (919.7.63.c.g.d.m)

920. The answer is d. (920.7.71.72.c.g.d.m)

921. The answer is d. (921.7.c.g.d.m)

922. The answer is b. (922.7.63.c.g.d.m)

923. The answer is d. (923.7.71.72.c.g.d.m)

924. The answer is d. (924.7.71.72.c.g.d.m)

925. The answer is c. (925.7.71.72.c.g.d.m)

926. The answer is a. (926.27.82.c.g.d.m)

927. The answer is c. (927.7.c.g.d.m)

928. The answer is a. (928.7.c.g.d.m)

929. The answer is d. (929.7.c.g.d.m)

930. The answer is a. Each of the other factors listed facilitate the care of the potentially suicidal patient and do not complicate the assessment. (930.38.c.g.d.m)

931. The answer is c. Fifty percent of completed suicides are associated with major depression. (931.10.12.13.15.25.38.c.g.d.m)

932. The answer is c. Approximately 10% of completed suicides are associated with schizophrenia and up to 10% of patients with schizophrenia will commit suicide. (932.12.38.63.c.g.d.m)

933. The answer is e. Approximately 50% of completed suicides are a result of affective illness and 15% of those with severe mood disorders will commit suicide. (933.13.14.38.63.c.g.d.m)

934. The answer is d. Approximately 25% of suicides are a result of alcoholism and drug dependence, often related to disinhibition and comorbid mood disorders. (934.12.38.63.c.g.d.m)

935. The answer is e. The lowest risk of suicide is found among those who are married. (935.38.63.c.g.d.m)

936. The answer is c. Panic disorder has recently been found to be an independent risk factor for suicide. (936.15.38.63.c.g.d.m)

937. The answer is d. For many individuals who make an impulsive attempt, once the impulse has been discharged, the individual's level of risk returns to baseline. (937.38.63.c.g.t.m)

938. The answer is a. When in doubt, be conservative and protect the patient from potential harm. Practice medicine like a physician, not like an attorney. (938.38.39.40.c.g.t.m)

939. The answer is b. Protection of the patient is required; after that, other information may be obtained. (939.38.39.40.44.c.g.t.m)

940. The answer is e. Protection of the patient may involve sitters, restraints, avoidance of harm, and escape. Rarely does it involve a benzodiazepine for sedation per se. (940.38.c.g.t.m)

941. The answer is d. While knowledge of plan may be useful during the evaluation, specific readings rarely are asked about. The means and details of a plan are important as areas of information together. (941.38.c.g.d.m)

942. The answer is d. Clinical factors (e.g., precipitants, plans for the future, disappointment about survival) are each more important than how health care will be reimbursed. (942.38.67.c.g.t.m)

943. The answer is e. HIV infection, psychosis, chronic renal failure, and stroke are all associated with suicide. Pancreatitis, while it may be associated with substance abuse and delirium, is not a known risk factor for suicide. (943.38.44.c.g.d.m)

944. The answer is c. Emotional reactions (e.g., anger and guilt) to a suicide are common and important. They should be discussed with colleagues and placed in perspective so as not to alter practice patterns adversely in the future. (944.38.68.c.g.d.m)

945. The answer is c. For men and women, the use of firearms is the most common method of completed suicide. (945.38.63.c.g.d.m)

946. The answer is b. In the Unites States, Caucasians suicide more often than do African-Americans. Women make more suicide attempts than men, and suicide rates increase as age increases. (946.38.63.c.g.d.m)

947. The answer is c. Approximately 15% of patients with major depression die by suicide. (947.13.38.63.c.g.d.m)

948. The answer is b. (948.38.63.c.g.d.m)

949. The answer is d. (949.38.63.c.g.d.m)

950. The answer is a. The same criteria used to diagnose major depression in the non–medically ill should be used in the medically ill. Level of oxygenation, presence of disorientation, myoclonus, or results of a DST are not diagnostic features of depression. (950.13.37.44.c.g.d.m)

951. The answer is a. Left frontal strokes commonly lead to depression, followed by right parietal and right frontal area strokes. (951.13.44.72.77. c.g.d.m)

952. The answer is a. Aprosodias involving dysregulation of the tonality and rhythm of speech are caused by lesions in the right hemisphere in a distribution that corresponds to aphasias associated with lesions in the left hemisphere. (952.44.72.77.78.c.g.d.m)

953. The answer is e. ECT is the most effective treatment for mood disorders, successfully treating more than 90% of afflicted patients. (953.13. 31.43.56.57.c.g.p.t.m)

954. The answer is c. In general, sedation of antidepressants correlates with affinity for histamine-1 receptors. (954.28.31.c.g.p.t.m)

955. The answer is b. TCAs commonly have anticholinergic effects and cause orthostatic hypotension and conduction system disturbances. (955. 31.35.36.c.g.p.t.m)

956. The answer is b. TCA-induced orthostatic hypotension is common but does not increase in the face of conduction system disturbance, while orthostatic hypotension secondary to MAOIs can be treated by cubes of cheddar cheese; TCA-induced orthostatic hypotension cannot. (956.31. 35.36.c.g.p.t.m)

957. The answer is c. The least anticholinergic of the agents listed is trazodone. Therefore, it would be least likely to cause urinary retention secondary to prostatic obstruction in elderly men. (957.31.35.36.44.c.g.p.t.m)

958. The answer is d. Of the agents listed, the SSRI, paroxetine, is the most anticholinergic. MAOIs, bupropion, and the benzodiazepine, alprazolam, are essentially nonanticholinergic. (958.28.29.31.c.g.p.t.m)

959. The answer is b. TCAs are associated with prolongation of the PR, QRS, and QTc as well as with sinus tachycardia. (959.31.36.84.c.g.p.t.m)

960. The answer is b. TCAs can worsen bundle branch blocks and lead to complete heart block, while ventricular ectopic activity could increase with the quinidine-like action of TCAs and atrial fibrillation could lead to 1-1 conduction in the ventricles in the presence of a TCA. (960.31. 36.44.84.c.g.p.t.m)

961. The answer is d. Nortriptyline, with a narrow therapeutic window, has reliable blood levels that correlate with response to treatment. (961.31.84.c.g.p.t.m)

962. The answer is a. While hypertension, decreased sleep, tachycardia, and cardiac arrhythmias are common with use of psychostimulants, anorexia is not a common side-effect. Instead, psychostimulants tend to increase, not decrease, appetite. (962.34.36.44.c.g.p.t.m)

963. The answer is e. Lithium is not associated with prolongation of the QRS complex, but it is associated with other electrocardiographic changes. (963.32.36.84.c.g.p.t.m)

964. The answer is d. Symptoms of dysthymia are the same as those of depression. In neither case is mood lability a diagnostic feature. (964.13.c. g.d.m)

965. The answer is e. Hypochondriasis is not managed with ECT, but instead with frequent visits by the PCP and with supportive care. (965. 12.13.14.43.79.c.g.t.m)

966. The answer is c. Catatonia, often with immobility, leads to decubitus ulcers, pneumonia, contractures, and pulmonary emboli, but not seizures. (966.44.79.c.g.d.m)

967. The answer is d. (967.12.13.43.78.79.c.g.t.m)

968. The answer is d. (968.43.74.79.c.g.t.m)

969. The answer is d. (969.43.c.g.t.m)

970. The answer is d. (970.43.c.g.t.m)

971. The answer is b. (971.43.c.g.t.m)

972. The answer is c. (972.43.c.g.t.m)

973. The answer is c. (973.43.c.g.t.m)

974. The answer is e. (974.43.c.g.t.m)

975. The answer is d. (975.13.43.63.c.g.t.m)

976. The answer is c. (976.13.43.63.c.g.t.m)

977. The answer is e. Experienced practitioners of ECT do not list any of these conditions as absolute contraindications to ECT. (977.43.44.63.c. g.t.m)

978. The answer is c. Cardiac outputs increase not decrease, and blood pressure increases and catecholamine increases, while parasympathetic tone remains strong. (978.43.c.g.t.m)

979. The answer is c. Beta-blockers often decrease the blood pressure, heart rate, and arrhythmias that follow ECT and are beneficial even in extremely high doses in cardiac patients undergoing ECT. (979.34.43. 44.c.g.t.m)

980. The answer is b. By contrast, lesions in Broca's area lead to nonfluent aphasia. (980.27.71.72.c.g.d.m)

981. The answer is b. Other structures thought to be part of the limbic system include the hippocampus, the amygdala, and the thalamus. (981. 27.72.c.g.d.m)

982. The answer is c. While many have studied the limbic system, it was Paul MacLean who coined the term. (982.27.72.c.g.d.m)

983. The answer is e. Each of the others are part of the language circuit. (983.27.71.72.c.g.d.m)

984. The answer is d. (984.12.27.c.g.d.m)

985. The answer is e. (985.27.72.c.g.d.m)

986. The answer is e. The insula is not part of the frontal lobe. (986.27.72.c.g.d.m)

987. The answer is c. Aprosodia is usually seen after a stroke in the right hemisphere. (987.27.71.72.c.g.d.m)

988. The answer is a. Executive function and judgment have been associated with frontal lobe development. (988.27.72.c.g.d.m)

989. The answer is d. The Svotchec sign is associated with calcium dysregulation. (989.27.71.72.c.g.d.m)

990. The answer is c. (990.27.72.c.g.d.m)

991. The answer is d. (991.27.72.c.g.d.m)

992. The answer is b. Nonfluent or expressive aphasias result from lesions in Broca's area near the motor strip. (992.27.71.72.c.g.d.m)

993. The answer is a. (993.27.71.72.c.g.d.m)

994. The answer is a. (994.27.71.72.c.g.d.m)

995. The answer is b. (995.27.71.72.c.g.d.m)

996. The answer is c. (996.79.c.g.d.m)

997. The answer is d. (997.79.c.g.d.m)

998. The answer is c. (998.79.c.g.d.m)

999. The answer is d. (999.79.c.g.p.d.t.m)

1000. The answer is d. (1000.6.44.c.g.p.d.m)

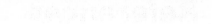

References

Samuels MA (ed): *Manual of Neurologic Therapeutics,* 5/e. Boston, Little Brown, 1994.

Stern TA, Herman JB (eds): *Massachusetts General Hospital Psychiatry Update and Board Preparation,* 2/e. New York, McGraw-Hill, 2004.

Stern TA, Herman JB, Slavin PL (eds): *The MGH Guide to Psychiatry in Primary Care.* New York, McGraw-Hill, 1998.

Stern TA, Herman JB, Slavin PL (eds): *The MGH Guide to Primary Care Psychiatry,* 2/e. New York, McGraw-Hill, 2004.